I H

Neil A

IS

978-1

ISBN-10:

1502475316

CW00385007

INTRODUCTION

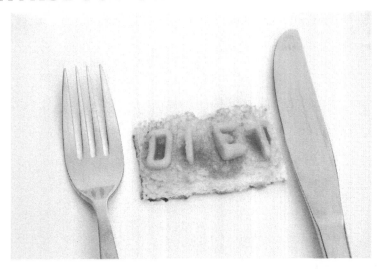

© Depositphotos.com/griffin024

I did ponder the title of this book and came up with a few ideas. I settled on "I Hate Diets" for a few reasons. The first reason is that I do actually hate diets, I don't like what they stand for a think that the word "Diet" has been hijacked by people trying to cash in on unsustainable strategies for losing weight. Diet has become a synonym for "Temporary" and "Trend". Saying that you are "Going on a diet" could easily be rewritten as "I'm going to follow the trend for a bit until I can't keep it going any longer or it's no longer in fashion".

Saying that you are "Going on a diet" could easily be rewritten as "I'm going to follow the trend for a bit until I can't keep it going any longer or it's no longer in fashion". Do you want temporary success or permanent success? Your diet, in the true meaning of the word, is something that you always have, it's your way of life.

Your diet is your way of eating and drinking. It's like religion, not just for Sundays, or football, not just Saturday afternoons; your diet is a permanent entity that will help define you; figuratively and literally. I also am against diets because of what clients and other people have told me.

They hate diets. How do you feel about them? I've heard so many stories about people hating the diet that they're on yet they desperately try and stick with it only to give it up after a few weeks, days or even hours! Have you ever had that?

The whole concept is wrong and the aim appears to be a mechanic selling you a flat tyre. You'll be OK for a bit, but sooner or later it's going to fail and you'll be back for another. He wouldn't want to sell you a good tyre from the beginning or you might never come back. He needs to make sure you will come back.

The same is true of the diet, if they all did what they say, everyone would only ever diet once! All studies relating to successful weight loss paint a grim picture and all studies relating to weight maintenance give an even grimmer picture.

Bearing in mind a success constitutes keeping only 5% of the weight lost off for a year, the number of people who were obese but are now a healthy weight is pretty small.

I attribute this to the methods people use, which in

most cases is some kind of diet. The list below has been compiled with my experience and those of my clients, to whom I have served as a weight loss helper.

I hope they can help you as well by preventing you from the same negative experiences.

Diets Deprive You

Most diets deprive you from eating what you want to eat.

They do this in two ways.

Way 1 - they tell you that you can't eat certain foods. It's just human nature that being told you're not allowed to eat something means that you suddenly want to eat it more than you did before. It's not uncommon to eventually give in to the obsession, eat what you shouldn't, feel guilty about eating it and eat a bit more to deal with the guilt. How about that for a vicious cycle?!

This feeling of deprivation is de-motivating and the diet ends there.

Way 2 - they give you a ridiculously low amount of food for the day. Diets that give you a miniscule amount of calories per day. A 30 year old woman, who is 1.55m tall and weighs 60 kilograms needs roughly 1,375 calories per day just to lay in bed and do nothing. Your brain, heart, liver and the rest of your organs need calories just to keep you alive. If you get up and walk around, do exercise and lead a busy life you'll obviously use more. These 850 calorie a day diets are totally unsuitable and in some cases can be dangerous. Weight loss is not about deprivation and healthy weight loss certainly isn't about deprivation!

Don't give yourself more problems, any diet that drastically reduces your calories should be avoided.

Diets Don't Give You an Exit Strategy

When you have lost weight on your given choice of diet, your options are to go one of two ways. The first way you can do is to keep doing the diet, which, if it's shakes, ready meals, calorie counting, food excluding etc. means doing that forever. The second option is to go back to what you were doing before and therefore put the weight on. Neither option is a good option in my book.

Diets are designed to fail so that keep returning to them and the people behind the diet can keep making money from you. A large and well known weekly weigh in group in America have a lifetime membership option. Some people may want to go to a weekly weigh in and eat weight loss club branded food for the rest of their lives, but you have to ask yourself that question. You need to find out how you're going to maintain that weight in a way that works for you.

Diets Make False Promises

Not losing weight fast enough can be a source of frustration. I get it, I do, I've been there. Worst is the weeks where you don't lose any at all! The human body is immensely complicated and there are thousands of things that influence how fast you lose or gain weight.

4

No one really fully understands the whole process. And to make it worse, it's different for everyone. Your genes, your body shape, your gender, your metabolism, your activity levels, what you eat and lots of other things can affect your weight. Not everyone will lose weight at the same rate even if they eat or do the same things. The more gradual your weight loss, the more chance there is of that weight not coming back. Expectations can be altered by TV programmes like the Biggest Loser.

It's important to remember the big reality weight loss show and weight loss won't be as drastic as the 41lbs in one week that is the current record. A healthy and sustainable weight loss amount is 1-2lbs per week. So while it may seem like it is taking an age, changing your diet and lifestyle is having a greater impact than just losing 1-2lbs a week.

That's enough about what this book is not and why it's not about dieting What this book does contain is a blueprint for changing various aspects of your lifestyle to give yourself the best possible chance of meeting your goals. If you can relate to any of those reasons above, then you will get lots out of this book.

Implement none of it, and you'll see no difference. Implement 50% of it, and you'll see a difference. Implement 90% of it and bingo, you're going to have great success.

Diets Don't Work With You

You're a unique person and you have your own personality, your own job, your own circumstances, your own likes and dislikes and your own family life. There is no one diet out there that can work for everyone. Diets are generally a set of rules, to which you should adhere or the whole thing falls apart.

Your diet needs to work with you and in order to work with you it needs to be flexible. Diets out there today just aren't flexible. What works for you might not work for someone else. Diets don't take this into account, they just tell you what to do and expect sheer willpower to get you through. Humans just aren't like that, I know I'm not and I am guessing you aren't, either.

In Closing

I believe in everything that is in this book and I know you will get a lot of out it. Just by reading this far, you're taking important steps to lasting change.

And that's the whole point, I want you to not only change the next week of your life, but the next six months and the next six years and beyond!

I'm thrilled about your decision to lose weight and I'm eager to get you on your way, so enjoy the book and please do let me know how you get on. You can email me at neil@neilashbyweightloss.co.uk.

Positively supporting your success,

Neil.

Chapter 1

The Successful Weight Loss Mindset

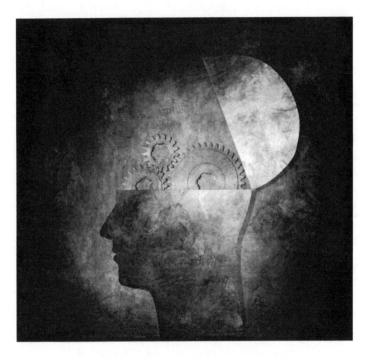

© Depositphotos.com/stocksnapper

So, you want to lose weight? That's the best thing you could have said today! I'm very happy for you that you want to lose some weight.

Are you serious about your weight loss? Do you realise the commitment that is required? Losing weight is not just a weekly class you can go to or something that takes five minutes a day, it's something that requires an ongoing commitment on a daily basis. You can't do it from a distance, you need to get in the action, confront it and stay in the game until you've achieved what you set out to achieve, even if it takes a while. Are you prepared for that?

How serious are you about losing weight? Give yourself a rating of how serious you are on a scale of 0-10. Why have you rated yourself at that level? If you aren't sure whether you are serious or if you are just casually wishing weight loss because you think you should, you definitely want to read this chapter.

The fact you are reading this is a positive sign and a step in the right direction, so you should feel pleased with that.

It may be fair to say that whatever actions have led you to this your current situation (and weight) will not lead you anywhere different if you continue on the same path. It is important to accept this point; **no change from you means no change in outcome**. More on that next chapter.

Mindset is an important part of any weight loss or weight management attempt. It may be fair to say that you have had previous attempts to lose weight and that these have been unsuccessful. What's your mindset like right now?

- Are you tired of trying to lose weight?
- Are you demoralised with the constant yo-yo cycle of dieting?
- Are you feeling more desperate as time goes on?

I understand how repeatedly trying something and not succeeding takes its toll on your gas tank, every attempt feels harder than the last and it gets more difficult to stick at something as time goes on. The diet is less fun than staying the same weight. There must be a better way!

One reason why the weight loss and weight management methods I coach people in are successful is because they are sustainable and not a temporary change.

There is a difference between a temporary diet and a permanent change and the mindsets associated with each are different. When you are making big decision in your life, perhaps you are thinking about a new job, new hobby, new partner etc., you should ask yourself, "Is this going to be a long term gig"? If it's only short term, what would be the point? In regards to weight loss, short term changes may work but with regards to weight management over a number of years, short term changes are not the way to go. We're looking at weight loss and successful weight management for the rest of your life, not a repeating cycle of short term weight loss, followed by weight regain. So, what you are going to do needs to be something you can do for years.

There is a man in Wiltshire who celebrates Christmas every day with a full Christmas dinner, mince pies and self addressed cards and has done for over 18 years.

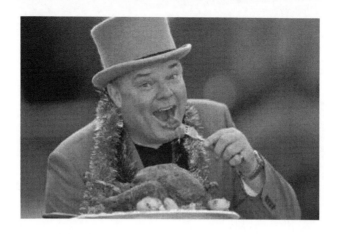

Andy Park he clearly loves it, he acknowledges he's had copycats but they just can't stick at it like he can. He's obviously a unique person!

I don't think that expecting you to stick to such a repetitive and restrictive regime is a realistic thing to expect of you. It is unlikely that anyone is going to adhere to a diet for the rest of their lives, whether it's the Christmas Dinner diet or a three shakes a day diet. It's just not realistic, not healthy and it's certainly not enjoyable (although with the Christmas Dinner approach you do get presents every day).

I am sure that some people are on various diets and points systems for years, but I think it is safe to say that the majority of us would prefer an alternative method to attaining a healthy weight.

It's been said that the best diet is the one you do not know you are on; and that is handy, because I don't want you to go on a diet. Below are some of the differences between the mindset that is geared towards dieting and one that is geared towards sustainability.

Issue	Diet Mindset	Sustainable Mindset
Goal	Weight Loss	Freedom and confidence in ability to make choices
Food	Food is the enemy	Food is food, nourishment, neither good nor bad
Attitude	Perfectionist	Flexible, go with the flow
Hunger	Eat when diet says so	In tune with body and internal cues
Unhealthy food	Bad	Just unhealthy
Quantity	Restrict/avoid	Moderation and balance
Eating	Deprivation / guilt	Enjoyment

My approach is one that leads to slower weight loss than other extreme forms but my approach leads to permanent weight loss and sustainable eating habits.

It's also an approach that is great for families and will set good examples to children. Some diets out there are not family friendly, such as the 3 shakes a day diet, the starve yourself for 2 days diet or the get food in packets delivered to your door each week diet. It's not as if any child is going to learn good habits from that day after day. These diets separate you from your family at mealtimes, which can send mixed and confusing messages to your children, and, again, it's not sustainable. I don't think it's useful for children to think that they can't be a healthy weight unless they replace food with shakes, eat less than 500 calories for two days a week or open dried food from a packet for their evening meal.

What I'm going to help you do is make a change in your values, a change in your habits and guide you towards permanent weight loss - no more diets. How does that sound?

Reasons to change

You will already know why you are thinking about losing weight. You'll have your reasons and your personal motivators. I want you to be thinking about these when reading the next section because it's often the negative and defeatist voice in us that shouts loudest.

Reasons not to change

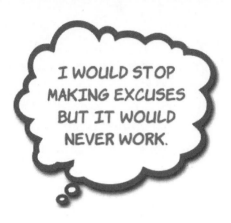

If the above sounds good and you've got plenty of reasons to change, skip this section. If you have already begun thinking about reasons why what I have said will not work or that it sounds good for other people but will not work for you, keep reading.

I don't like the word "excuse", I have to say, because I think there is a stigma attached to it. I'm going to give you the benefit of the doubt and not really consider your possible objections as excuses, I will call them concerns.

Excuses are for people trying to get out of something, concerns are for people who want to do it but they see some potential barriers.

I want to take a few moments to remove all the barriers to your weight loss. Whatever concerns you may have, we can deal with them and pass safely on round them.

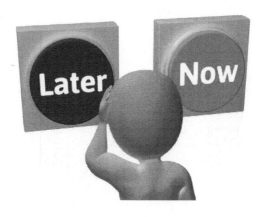

Are any of these what you are thinking as reasons why you can't achieve your weight loss and successful weight management over the long term? Tick the ones that you have used before or still believe now.

☐ My job gets in the way

☐ I never have enough time

☐ I have a busy family life

☐ The children make it difficult

☐ I don't have much disposable income

☐ I can start this next week

☐ I have a low metabolism

☐ I have a medical condition so losing weight is really

difficult

☐ I haven't exercised in years

☐ I am addicted to some foods

☐ I don't like new foods

☐ I have no one to help me

☐ I don't like to go outside when it rains

☐ I can't afford healthy food

☐ I put on weight really easily

☐ I can never do it, I've failed before

☐ I am scared of failure

☐ I am scared of criticism

☐ I am embarrassed to leave the house

☐ I have missed my chance

☐ I am just unlucky

☐ I don't know how

☐ I don't have the willpower

☐ I can't stick at this

☐ I find losing weight too difficult

☐ I am not meant to lose weight

☐ I don't know where to start

☐ I quit things easily

These are some of the things you might be thinking and you might have said in the past about previous weight loss attempts.

I accept none of these statements. Not one. You shouldn't, either. I don't want you to allow those statements to come between you and your healthy weight and all the fantastic things that come with that. Are you defeated that easily? Accepting these excuses is not taking responsibility and accepting that you are in control of your actions and your actions are what determine your outcomes.

The reason that I do not accept any of these statements are true is that they are not helpful, they only serve to keep you where you are and not progress yourself in life. You may have a busy life, have a demanding job or have low willpower but that does not mean you can't be a healthy weight. How many barriers have you faced in life? I am sure there have been lots, but yet you still achieved what you set out to do. If you want to use these false beliefs to justify why you can't lose weight, then that's OK but that's not the mindset of someone who is going to succeed.

If it allows you to sleep easy and allows you to accept

your weight because you are too busy to be a healthy weight, that's OK, but it's not the mindset of someone who is going to succeed.

If you look at everyone who has successfully maintained a healthy weight, whether they've lost weight or not, and think that none of these people have any of the same barriers you do or have it as hard as you do, that's fine, if it allows you to accept your weight and carry on without change, but it's not the mindset of someone who is going to succeed.

The only statements I will accept that will prevent you from losing weight are:

• I do not believe I should lose weight

• I do not believe I can lose weight

I call these the Terrible Two because other than being terrible and there being two of them, they both need banishing if you want success. I am going to deal with both of those right now, because without a big NO to both statements, weight loss is not going to happen.

I do not believe I should lose weight

If you don't think you need to lose weight then you're

simply not going to. Some people aren't sure if they need to or not, others never really think about it because they know the truth but can't face the reality of where they are. If you don't think you should lose weight or you simply don't want to, please read on below.

The first step is to see where your weight falls on the chart below. This chart is based on your Body Mass Index (BMI), which gives you a score based on your height and weight. Your score determines whether you are classed as under weight, a healthy weight, over weight, obese or morbidly obese. Plot your height and weight on the chart below and see which category you fall into.

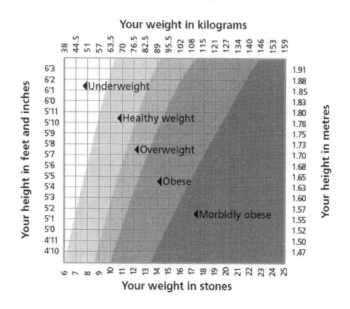

BMI is a good standard but does not take into account

your body build, your genetic make up or your activity level.

A good indicator of whether or not you should be looking at weight loss is your waist size. This, combined with the BMI result provides a clearer picture of your risk of health issues due to your weight. The table below shows the waist measurements and their associated risk levels.

Waist Circumference M = male F = female	BMI Classification		
	Healthy weight	Over-weight	Obese
Low M: < 94cm / 37in F: < 80cm / 31.5in	No increased risk	No increased risk	Increased risk
High M: 94cm - 102cm F: 80cm - 88cm	No increased risk	Increased risk	High risk

Very High			
M: > 102cm / 40in F: > 88cm / 34.5in	Increased risk	High risk	Very high risk

I'm briefly going to mention some information about the health risks of obesity[1]. This information is taken from http://www.patient.co.uk. The diagram below is an overview of parts of the body affected by obesity and gives the common afflictions brought on by obesity or made worse by obesity.

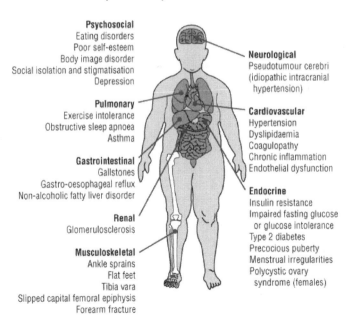

Psychosocial
Eating disorders
Poor self-esteem
Body image disorder
Social isolation and stigmatisation
Depression

Pulmonary
Exercise intolerance
Obstructive sleep apnoea
Asthma

Gastrointestinal
Gallstones
Gastro-oesophageal reflux
Non-alcoholic fatty liver disorder

Renal
Glomerulosclerosis

Musculoskeletal
Ankle sprains
Flat feet
Tibia vara
Slipped capital femoral epiphysis
Forearm fracture

Neurological
Pseudotumour cerebri
(idiopathic intracranial
hypertension)

Cardiovascular
Hypertension
Dyslipidaemia
Coagulopathy
Chronic inflammation
Endothelial dysfunction

Endocrine
Insulin resistance
Impaired fasting glucose
or glucose intolerance
Type 2 diabetes
Precocious puberty
Menstrual irregularities
Polycystic ovary
syndrome (females)

If you are overweight or obese, from day to day you may:

• Feel tired and lacking in energy

• Experience breathing problems (for example, shortness of breath when moving around, or not being able to cope with sudden bursts of physical activity like running across the road)

• Feel that you sweat a lot compared with other people

• Develop skin irritation

• Have difficulty sleeping

• Get complaints from your partner that you snore.

• Experience back and joint pains which can affect your mobility.

You may also have an increased risk of developing:

• Impaired glucose tolerance (pre-diabetes)

• Type 2 diabetes

• High cholesterol or triglyceride levels.

• High blood pressure

• Coronary heart disease

- Stroke

- Sleep apnoea (this is when your breathing patterns are disturbed while you are sleeping, due to excess weight around your chest, neck and airways)

- Fertility problems

- Complications in pregnancy (including an increased risk of high blood pressure during pregnancy, diabetes during pregnancy, preterm labour, caesarean section)

- Stress incontinence (leaking urine when you are, for example, laughing, coughing, etc)

- Gallstones

- Cancers (including colon, breast and endometrial (womb) cancer)

- Gout

- Fatty liver

Many people can also develop psychological problems because of being overweight or obese. For example: low self-esteem; poor self-image (not liking how you look); low confidence; feelings of isolation. These feelings may affect your relationships with family members and friends and, if they become severe, may lead to depression.

Being obese can also affect your overall life expectancy[2]: you are more likely to die at a younger age. An analysis in 2009 of almost one million people from around the world showed that if you have a BMI between 30 and 35, you are likely to die 2-4 years earlier than average. If your BMI is between 40 to 45, you are likely to die 8-10 years earlier than average.

Another analysis showed that if you are a woman who is obese at the age of 40, you are likely to die 7.1 years earlier than average. If you are a man who is obese at the age of 40, you are likely to die 5.8 years earlier than average. It's easy to ignore these figures but there is real information behind them.

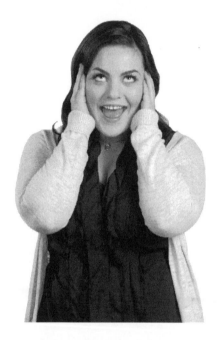

© Depositphotos.com/creatista

Even a modest amount of weight loss can help conditions caused by obesity. Some conditions are cured altogether so it's well worth losing weight if you are overweight or obese.

How do you feel about losing weight now? Is it something that you believe you should do and something that you want to do? The answer needs to be yes, just like any other accomplishment or goal, to achieve success, you the necessary motivation or want.

Let us now discuss the second of the Terrible Two beliefs.

I do not believe I can lose weight

Henry Ford, the great American industrialist once said "Whether you believe you can, or whether you believe you can't; either way, you're right."

If you don't believe you can achieve something, what's point in even trying? This is why this member of the Terrible Two will put an end to your weight loss efforts before you have begun. It's important that you believe in yourself and have faith that you can achieve what you want to achieve.

I want you to write down your three biggest accomplishments. And spend time on this, think about them, enjoy the memory of accomplishing what you have, it will make the exercise more beneficial.

I then want you to write down the qualities that you needed to achieve those accomplishments.

I want you to write down your three best qualities, they can be anything.

I want you to imagine you are a friend, colleague, family member of yourself and write down what they would say your three best qualities are.

Now I want you to say aloud the following: "My name is <your name>, and I have accomplished the following: <list three accomplishments>. I accomplished these things because I am <list x qualities> and because I possess all of these qualities, I know I can accomplish my goal of being a healthy weight."

So, you could have said something like this "My name is Joe Bloggs and I have accomplished the following: completed a degree in science, raised 2 children and raised £500 for charity. I accomplished these things because I am caring, determined, hard working, funny, patient and devoted and because I possess all of these qualities, I know I can accomplish my goal of being a healthy weight."

Did you say it aloud or did you say it in your head? Say it aloud, no one can hear you, and say it like you mean it. If you can't even say it, how are you going to do it?

How does that sound? Do you now realise that you have what it takes? Given your amazing accomplishments and your excellent personal qualities, what do you think your chances are of losing weight and maintaining a health weight in the long term? I think they are excellent! If you still don't believe me, tell some of your friends that you want to lose weight and ask them if they believe in you. This might help you believe in yourself rather than believe that weight loss will control you in some way.

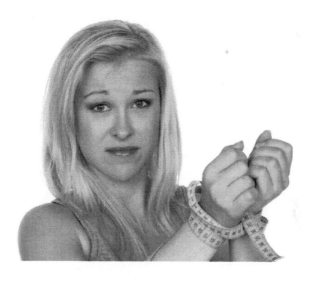

© Depositphotos.com/ginasanders

Now I have talked about the mindset you need for making changes and in this case, changes that support a healthy weight in the long term. You have rejected any false beliefs you hold as will come between you and success in anything, including losing weight. I've talked about the Terrible Two that will stop your weight loss efforts in their tracks. "I don't want to lose weight" and "I don't think I can lose weight" are going to kill your weight loss efforts stone dead. I have given you some health risks associated with obesity as well as other reasons why weight loss might be a good idea for you. I have also asked you to think about your accomplishments and qualities to prove to yourself that you absolutely can lose weight and maintain a healthy weight for the future.

So now I'm hoping that you have ticks against the following:

✓ I need to lose weight

✓ I want to lose weight

✓ I believe I can and will lose weight

Some people may not think that need to lose weight, despite their BMI or waist measurements. If you are in doubt, please visit your GP for further advice about whether weight loss will bring benefits.

When I coach people, I like to spend time talking about your motivation and what your thoughts are about weight loss. I also spend time helping you to prepare for what is ahead, which I've found to be an important aspect of successful weight loss.

If you are still struggling with one of the areas above, you can contact me and I'll be happy to discuss things with you.

When mountaineers talk about a successful climb, they say that in order to complete a successful climb, you must reach the summit and come down again, safely.

When I talk about successful weight loss, I'm do not only mean losing x amount of stones. I mean "Achieving your target weight, which is in the healthy range for your gender and height and maintaining this weight for at least five years while living a healthy lifestyle".

I want to highlight some statistics that stand out as important when we're talking about weight loss and weight management in the long term:

- 90-95% of people who go on a diet will regain at least the amount of weight they lost within three years[3]

- The average time spent on a diet is 5½ weeks, although in the North West, the average time is four days[4]

- The average woman diets twice a year and if dieting for seven weeks a year, this amounts to 17 years over her adult life[5]

These statistics don't tell an encouraging story in terms of the average weight loss experience. They say that you either lose weight and put it all back on again or you give up making changes after 37 days. I know you're not an average person, but do those sound like statements you would like to associate with yourself?

Do you want to lose weight and then put it all back on and more within three years? Do you want to find yourself three years down the line, feeling even worse than you did before? Do you want to spend 37 days on a diet and then 37 days on another diet and go through diets like shoes? I did not think so, and the good news is you don't need to.

You've ticked those boxes to say you need to lose weight, you want to lose weight and you believe you can lose weight, which is a fantastic start! Change is an important part of successful weight loss and that's what I'm going to talk about in the next chapter.

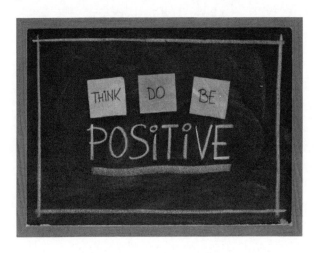

© Depositphotos.com/PixelsAway

Conclusion

Weight loss, change and commitment are all serious business. This is not something to enter into lightly, it's important to get your mindset right before beginning

- You need to know what it is that you want to do and why you are doing it. If you don't know what you want or why you want it, it's unlikely you'll succeed in getting it!
- You can have excuses or results, you can't have both. You are going to have results!

Chapter 2

Successful Approaches to Change

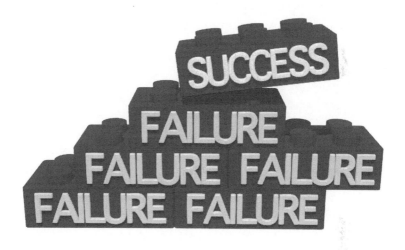

Change is defined as:

a. to make different in some particular : alter

b. to make radically different : transform

c. to give a different position, course, or direction to

Think about when the last time you made a change to something important in your life? When was the last time you did something for the first time? Change is not something that comes naturally to us and not something we generally embrace. Most of us don't change unless it is forced upon us and usually then it can involve feet dragging and a bit of grumbling.

Every workplace I've ever worked in has avoided change until the very last minute possible. When a new system was introduced, the old one was still used until it was physically withdrawn, when we had a deadline by which to pack our desks for office moves, we left it right until the last minute to move. It wasn't because we were lazy, we just didn't want change, we wanted things to continue how they were because it is comfortable, it's safe and it's familiar. The only time I ever changed promptly and without question was when it had anything to do with overtime and money and my lack of cooperation would have resulted in me not getting paid on time. When it was to do with getting paid, my cooperation was as forthcoming as perfume sellers in a department store.

By the end of this chapter, I want you do recognise that you will need to make changes and embrace this concept. I'm hoping that even if you are a bit sceptical of change and not really a fan of getting out of your comfort zone, you're mindset will be one of positivity, determination and a willingness to try new things. Think about the reasons you want to lose weight, all of them. In fact, write them down in a list and then write why each one is important to you.

Now you've written down all the reasons why you want to lose weight and why they're important to you, what do you think about them? They should be pretty powerful when you read them back to back to yourself.

When I work with my coaching clients, I spend a lot of time talking with them about change and motivation to get them ready for what's ahead.

Look at how fast I adapted to the new overtime form so I could make sure my overtime was paid, your reasons are a hundred times more important than my overtime so I would imagine that after writing your list of motivators, you can't wait to get started!

You want to change your weight, but that's not really the thing you're going to change. You can't just reduce your weight because your weight is the outcome. You need to change those things that affect the outcome. A simple change equation looks like this:

INPUT + PROCESS = OUTCOME

In other words "The stuff you have" + "What you do with it" = "Some kind of result".

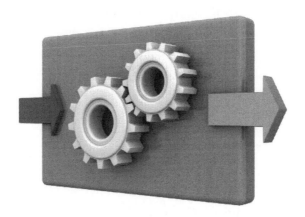

So we can't just go from unhealthy weight to healthy weight in an instant because the outcome is on the wrong side of the equals sign for us to be able to change it. What we need to do is change either the input or the process, the outcome will then follow.

You might be thinking that the above sounds difficult, a bit too much like hard work and wondering if there is another way. How about changing nothing but still having a different outcome? That would be something but it doesn't add up, that's why it's not possible. Wouldn't it be easier if there was a magic pill, an operation, a super shake or a 5 minute thinning booth each day that would make sure you stayed at a healthy weight? If the amount of effort and time that people put into pursuing these panaceas was put into other methods of change, their goal would already be achieved. Unfortunately, all time asking "What if?" is not far from "I want the easier way".

If someone spends their time searching for the super magic pill rather than actively changing, you could rewrite their equation like so:

No change + No change = NO CHANGE!

In the last chapter, I talked about some statistics regarding the success of diets, how long the average diet lasts and how long people on diets in their lifetime. None of the statistics were indicative of success. There are, of course, reasons for this.

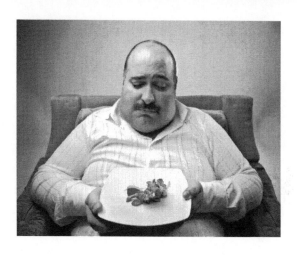

© Depositphotos.com/olly18

The fact that the average diet doesn't last more than 6 weeks is because people are unable to stick to it for longer than that. They want to lose weight, they really do, but they are just unable to pursue beyond that 6 week duration. And even then, what chance of success? Who says 6 weeks is enough? Maybe it needs 2 months? Maybe it requires the rest of your life? There is one fact to be gained from this information and that is simply that most weight loss attempts through going on a diet are doomed to fail before they have begun. This is a good example of changing the process to alter the outcome. The problem is, the process they change to is not the correct one and so the outcome is the same, namely failure, frustration and unhappiness.

Having the wrong input or the wrong process is not going to give you the outcome you want. So thought needs to be given to what the right course of action is before you start down the path.

This is a good example of the vicious cycle that dieting can be. One diet doesn't work, spend a month on that, try another. There are countless diets out there, an ever increasing number, so trying a new one seems like a good idea. Evidence and experience show that this is not the case. What this does achieve, though, is satisfying yourself in your mind that you are making an attempt to lose weight. You might even know after a day or two that this won't be something you can keep up but at least when you next talk about your weight with a friend and they ask you what you are doing, you can honestly and sincerely tell them that you are trying.

I have a real problem with this approach because you're worth much more than a half hearted try just so you can appease your inner thoughts, your family or your doctor. You are not going to be a person who tries to be a healthy weight, you are going to be a person who makes changes and successfully achieves and maintains their healthy weight. I'm not settling for the trying approach, and neither should you.

Diet Cycling

I'm sure you've probably heard of the term "Yo-yo dieting". There are two versions of yo-yo dieting. The first is where the person goes on a diet, loses some weight and therefore stops dieting, the weight creeps back on, usually to a point where they are heavier than before, then they decide to diet again. The process then repeats itself. The second version is where the person goes on a diet, finds they are unable to stick to the diet, so they try another diet for a period of time, have a hard time adhering to that diet and then the process repeats until they give up.

The cycle of dieting is shown below. Does any of it seem familiar to you?

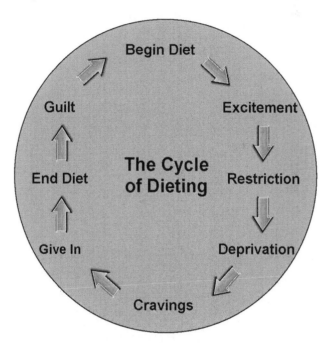

If you remember the 80s television series "Yes, Minister", about how the Civil Service tried to prevent politicians from making changes, you may be remember a saying from Arnold, the Cabinet Secretary. He was talking about how one of the Ministers, Jim Hacker, would want to change things because he thinks he ought to. Arnold's view, as well as the view of the Civil Service, is to do nothing, change is not something to be encouraged. Arnold mentioned "Politician's Logic" and it went along the lines of "I must do something, this is something, therefore I must do this".

I believe a similar thought process is prevalent in today's society and that's Dieter's Logic. This is where a person would like to lose weight and to them this means a diet and they'll seek out the latest high profile diet. "I need to lose weight, this is a diet, therefore I must go on this diet". While I think you and I both agree change is needed, making the right change is very different from making any old change.

I am sure you are familiar with the phrase "Fail to prepare; prepare to fail", which is what my dad taught me about DIY when I was growing up. Like any teenager who knows it all, I obviously didn't believe him and disregarded everything he said; his experience and knowledge counting for nothing. Clearly my best course of action was to carry on regardless. I would try and drill holes without measuring up and attempt to do it all by eye, only to realise the holes weren't straight and didn't line up with the picture I was hanging up. So then I had to do it all again and I was starting from a worse position than before. So a lot of time and energy wasted and me feeling foolish, somewhat deservedly, I must admit.

The analogy can be used with dieting. You rush into one diet because you feel compelled to act, don't really plan anything or think about the consequences, find it's not working for you, stop, realise you can't go on as you were and then come to a grinding halt. You then are either mentally defeated, you've maybe put on weight or you are more frustrated than you were before.

So, in terms of our equation earlier (Input + Process = Output), it's crucial that we get the right process. So when you have decided to take action and make a change, you may as well make the correct change, I talk about these in the next few chapters.

The Miracle Diet

When a new diet gets mainstream attention, people flock to it as if it were their saviour, the one they've been waiting for their entire diet ridden lives. Something new to try gives them hope, which is understandable, but as every new diet advertises itself as "THE diet, the one that REALLY works", an impartial observer might not be too convinced. I personally think it's bordering on cruel, it plays with people's emotions, gets their hopes up and often there's no real success or evidence behind the diets, just clever marketing and celebrities willing to put their names to it. There is a diet called "Juice Diet - lose 7lbs in 7 days", which is proving popular. I could lose 7lbs in 7 days, but what happens after the initial 7 days are up? Will I lose 7lbs every 7 days? Do I have to eat only juice for the rest of my life, I'd rather eat food. It's a complicated world out there for people who are looking to lose weight and maintain a healthy weight in a healthy way. People are bombarded with claims of diet miracles and images of chiselled people that are designed to hook us in and try to capture some of the dieting market. I think most of them are just unhelpful.

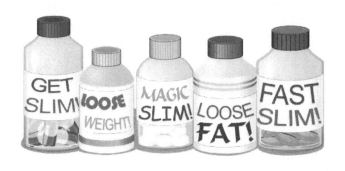

© Depositphotos.com/Mjak

As an example, the FAST diet, also known as the 5:2 diet and other names, has recently been given lots of attention. The FAST diet states that you consume no more than 500 calories on two days of the week and eat unrestricted amounts on the other 5 days. 3 of the top 5 books in Amazon's health section are on this subject 4 months after the launch and it's proved a very popular diet. One book had 4.5 stars out of 5 and had 1200 or so reviews, which is quite positive feedback. One reviewer, who gave it a 4 out of 5 said "Very interesting, definitely worth trying. I am on my second week of 5:2, it has been challenging so I am not sure how long I will last". So it might have the novelty factor, but is it something that is effective and sustainable? Are people doing it because it is successful for them or are they doing it because it's the next diet on the list?

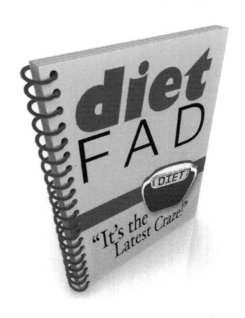

© Depositphotos.com/iqoncept

The Atkins diet burst onto the scene a few years ago and had 1 in 11 Americans on the diet.[1] That's over 20 million people! How many do you think are still on the diet? A year after it peaked, the Atkins Nutritional company filed for bankruptcy. If the Atkins diet was a long term successful approach to weight management, we wouldn't have had the Dukan Diet and if the Dukan Diet was so successful, we wouldn't have had the Fast Diet. In fact, as popular as the Dukan Diet was, The British Dietetic Association named in the top 5 diets to avoid for three years running[2]. I wonder if I could launch the "Poke yourself in the eye whilst eating" diet and people would give it a go simply because it got media attention. Well, maybe not, but you get the idea. The fact that the British Dietetic Association has to tell you to avoid them shows you how much momentum even an appalling diet can have when endorsed by a celebrity (Of course, Simon Cowell, Rhianna and Kate Moss are well renowned for their nutritional knowledge and healthy lifestyles). One thing you could do is go up to a celebrity who endorses a particular diet and ask them if their children are on that diet. The answer might tell you, and them, how sensible it really is or how crazy they really are.

Weight loss is too important to be darting about from one diet to another, your time and emotions are too valuable to be putting your energies into something that is almost certain to fail.

Apart from the obvious practical issues with adhering to one set of rules for 6 weeks, then adhering to a totally different set of rules for another 6 weeks, there are emotional implications as well. Trying desperately to stick to a diet, not getting the results you want and not really enjoying the process can leave you feeling grumpy, tired, frustrated down demotivated.

This may seem familiar to you but it is also the reality for a lot of other people. If you read what is asked of you on some of the diets, it's a wonder you can even function properly in today's society. For example, the Ketogenic Enteral Nutrition diet, or KEN diet means you don't eat anything.[3] Obviously a genius idea developed with the well being of the dieter in mind. Instead of eating food, you ingest a patented liquid formula made up of protein and nutrients, which is then dripped directly into the stomach via a plastic tube that goes up the dieter's nose and is taped on to their face (see picture below).

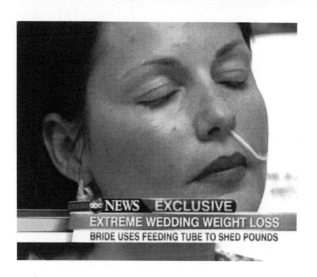

NEWS EXCLUSIVE
EXTREME WEDDING WEIGHT LOSS
BRIDE USES FEEDING TUBE TO SHED POUNDS

At the other end of the tube is an electric pump, which works constantly to deliver two litres of the formula over 24 hours. While on the KEN, dieters can go about their lives as normal but must carry the pump and liquid in a bag or backpack and hang it by their bed at night. They are allowed to unhook themselves from the pump for one hour a day (for bathing, showering etc.) and can drink water, tea, coffee (with no milk, sugar or sweeteners) or sugar-free herb teas with the tube.

Now, what circumstances could lead you to decide the KEN diet is for you? It's almost impossible to imagine but these are the lengths people will go to because they feel they have no other option. The sense of despair, unhappiness and the lack of support they are getting means they think this is a viable option. That's how big an issue this is for people. Part of the message I want to convey in this book is that there is another option, an alternative to the many diets out there. Clients I have worked with have tried all sorts of different diets, and even with all these diets, they still weren't successful in achieving their goals because those diets weren't meant for long term success; they were meant to make money.

Dealing with Setbacks

When changing aspects of your life, it is inevitable that you will find things difficult at some point. I want to talk about how to deal with setbacks because having a strategy for this now will be really useful over the coming weeks and months. The first thing to do is accept that setbacks happen, perhaps you put some weight on one week or maybe you had a couple more pints than you planned to have one night, things don't always go the way you would have wanted.

Setbacks will happen on your weight loss and weight management journey, this is without question and ignoring this fact will not be useful. Having the ability to recognise what they are and deal with them is crucial to preventing a setback from turning into a failure.

My Mum has been to a well known, national, weekly slimming club and every week they have a meeting, where the members are weighed. I will ask her how she got on and on some weeks she might say "Not very well, I've put on half a pound" and she'd be a little despondent about it. I don't know why this is classed as "Not very well" or what mindset the group had, but our weight fluctuates, this is not something recently discovered. But hydration levels, hormones, salt intake, food, recently going to the toilet and any recent exercise can all affect your weight. Weighing in at half a pound more than last week isn't something that should be classed as a setback and that should play on your mind.

This would only be something that can be classed as a setback if there's clearly weight to be lost and a slight weight gain is happening repeatedly over the course of a month. Trends over weeks and months should be going in the right direction but if for a couple of weeks you put on half a pound, it's nothing to despair over. Surely if someone has made some positive changes to their diet and to their lifestyle, this is something to be celebrated rather than ignored in favour of focusing on half a pound gained? That half a pound means nothing, positive changes are going to give you results for the rest of your life.

A setback is not going to turn your weight loss effort into a failure unless you allow it to, you are in control. If I am walking to the shops and I stumble and fall, I've had a setback. I still want to go to the shops, so I get up again and carry on, arriving slightly late but still achieving my goal. If I had chosen to stay on the floor and not get up, I would have not achieved my goal and that setback would have become a failure. I decided whether I got up or not, I was in control.

Setbacks can occur in many ways; events, occasions and places all have potential to create a setback. Perhaps a busy day at work, an invitation to a party, a meal at a restaurant or a family birthday. These all present the opportunity for a setback.

For every setback you have, I want you to recognise it for what it is, have a strategy for preventing it from becoming a failure and then implement that strategy this time and in future times. This will allow you to prevent the setback from occurring in the first place and allow you to recover more quickly from one that does occur.

What turns a setback into a failure? The answer to that is you and your attitude. There isn't a single thing that can turn a weight loss attempt into a failure, just as there is no single thing that can assure successful weight loss.

When a setback occurs, there can be a temptation to believe it represents total failure. You may think you are weak for letting something like that occur, or you may think that you can never succeed because this has happened. Clearly, neither of these are true, but it is a common initial reaction to the setback. The danger is that this will snowball into something much bigger. For example, if you've had one pint, you may as well have five, or you've had a biscuit so you may as well eat the entire packet or perhaps you have had a chocolate bar in the morning and then write off the entire day and pig out. These would be overreactions to what would essentially be a stumble and remember, you are not a professional footballer, when you stumble, you are going to get back to your feet and keep going.

Talking about the setbacks can help. When I coach clients I'll talk a lot about the potential for setbacks and how to deal with them. They find it very useful to talk about the stumbles and we talk about the strategies for dealing with them practically and mentally. This gives them more confidence when avoiding or recovering from a setback.

The Critical Five - CASES

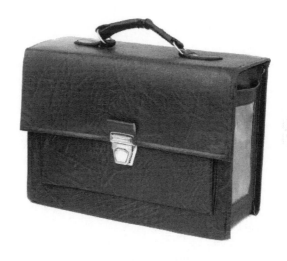

© Depositphotos.com/inarik

Remember the KEN diet? There are reasons why many people wouldn't do that. I bet you could come up with a few reasons now. When you want to assess whether something is a good idea, have a look below at the five criteria I've mentioned, easily remembered by the acronym CASES. When I work with clients, I only ask them to make changes that adhere to these five criteria. If they don't adhere to CASES, there's no point in doing them because you are looking to make the right changes, not just an old change. The criteria are:

- Comfortable

- Achievable

- Sustainable

- Effective

- Sensible

My reasons for why I think each of these belong in the Critical Five as below.

Comfortable - if you are not comfortable with something, you're not going to make that lasting change. For example, if I asked you to eat something you didn't like or do an activity you didn't enjoy, this wouldn't be something you were comfortable with so an alternative must be found.

Achievable - if something isn't achievable then there's not much point in spending time trying to achieve it. You won't get any benefit and you'll give up and feel bad, making further attempts more difficult. Note, there is a big difference between something not being achievable and you not believing that you can achieve it. For example, if I asked you to never eat chocolate again, this may not be achievable because you actually quite enjoy chocolate, so we'd talk about how to work around that.

Sustainable - surely what you do must be sustainable. If something isn't sustainable, then it's temporary. Do you want temporary or permanent weight loss? If your weight loss is attributed to something you can't do on a long term basis, the weight is going to come right back to you. For example, you may be able to eat meal replacement shakes and bars for a couple of weeks, but how about the rest of your life?

Sensible - Be sensible, my mother always says. Good advice, Mum. Why would you not want to do something that isn't sensible, especially when it is to do with your health? We want it to be practical, safe and reasonable. We also want it to not have any negative side effects on your health or the rest of your life. An example of something I wouldn't consider sensible would be the KEN diet.

Effective - you want to be doing something that works. This means it's worth your effort and your valuable time. If it doesn't work or works for only a short time, it's not much use to you. For example, diets that promise 7lbs in 7 days but after that, a slow regain of the 7lbs ensues.

So everything you change has to meet the CASES criteria, but what kind of things should you be changing? That's what we're going to discuss next.

Chapter 3

Create an Environment for Weight Loss

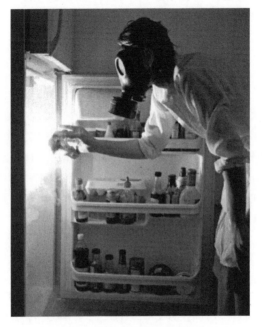

© Depositphotos.com/jhet45

Compare the houses of a couple with children and a couple without children. People with children generally have protectors on the plug sockets, barriers at the bottom and top of the stairs, a fire place screen, cupboard locks in the kitchen and anything remotely dangerous to a child will be put out of reach. Not to mention the toys and child paraphernalia that will no doubt be scattered everywhere throughout the house.

What's happening here is that the parents have altered

their environment to promote the task of bringing up children. I am sure not all of the changes are welcome, no more tidy house, no more space, always having to clear away anything unsafe for children and having to watch out for toy trains under your feet. Despite this, the changes are made and the parents raise their children.

You may have worked out why I am saying this, and it is because to achieve a goal, you need to give yourself the best possible chance of achieving this by engineering an environment to support your goal. Weight loss and weight management is similar to bringing up a child in the sense it's a big thing and it is a constant thing that takes place in the home, at work and in other locations.

In order to achieve your goal, you need to manage your environment to help you achieve this. Why would you continue to surround yourself in an environment that is detrimental to you achieving your goals? You wouldn't, you want to give yourself the best possible chance of losing weight initially and maintaining a healthy weight in the long term and just like charity, this starts in the home.

The Home

Your home environment is critical to any effort to achieve a healthy weight. Have a look around your house and make a mental note of all the objects that could have an affect on your health or on your weight.

This could be the layout of the rooms, the types of chairs you have, the amount of televisions you have, the way your garden is landscaped etc..

I'll give you a few common examples:

- Most people have the TV as the focal point of their living room and to watch TV you sit, slouch or lay down on a settee or arm chair. Why not lose the arm chair and replace it with an exercise bike or a Swiss ball? You can then watch TV while you are exercising or sitting with proper posture on the ball. The ball means you must use your core and you can even do some simple exercises whilst sitting on it.

- Have you a space in the garden for any form of exercise, games or activity? Could you rearrange things to create even a small amount of space?

- Do you have a TV in your bedroom? Does this encourage you to spend longer laying down rather than encouraging you to get up and get going with the day?

- How much clutter and mess is in your house? Can you find things easily? Can you do what you need to do without having to spend 10 minutes moving stuff about first and then spend another 10 minutes looking for what it is you need?

- There are those that keep a mini fridge in the living room or by the bed that contains beer, chocolate, fizzy drinks and the like. The only place food should be stored is in the kitchen.

- Can you eat at the table? Is your dining room table full of colouring books, the post, newspapers, computers, general clutter that you can't find a home for? This needs clearing so you can have a proper place to eat.

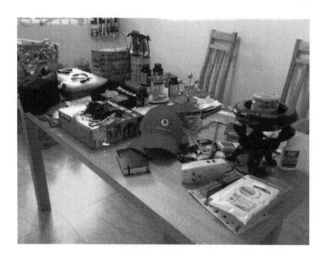

© Depositphotos.com/lashtat

Think about your house and whether it lends itself to supporting you and your healthy weight.

If you wanted to go for a walk now, would you be able to find your clothes easily? How about your walking shoes or trainers? A bottle of water to take with you? These things should be easy to get your hands on because in the time taken to organise it all, you can talk yourself out of it and not bother. I'm not saying you should tidy up ready for a royal visit, but you need to be able to minimise the effort it takes to prepare for exercise. Why would you make it hard for yourself? Why would you bury the bicycle under loads of stuff in the garage? You'll never bother to use it. You wouldn't throw your car keys across the room when you got home so you'd have a job to find them the next day when you go to work. You need to make it as easy as possible for yourself to do things that support a healthy lifestyle. So allowing yourself easy access to those things that help you achieve this is an important step.

There are other benefits to decluttering and making things tidy. You'll get a great sense of satisfaction, you'll have achieved something, you'll be getting some good exercise and you get a tidier home, which is much easier to live in!

I don't want to go on about this too much as there are many resources out there to help you plan a strategy for decluttering your house, but I want to stress the point that it is important to have a healthy home. You probably spend more time at home than anywhere else so the opportunities for not doing activity, increasing sedentary time or taking in extra calories are plentiful. By making changes, you are making it that little bit easier to achieving your healthy weight.

The Kitchen

I separate your kitchen from the rest of your home

because this is where the action is at. What does your kitchen say about you? How easy is it to cook in your kitchen? How is your fridge arranged? What's on the kitchen counter? What's in the cupboards?

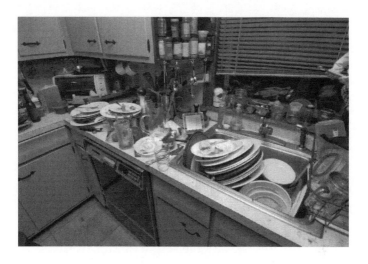

© Depositphotos.com/sonar

Let's take a closer look at each of these.

Cooking - cooking food yourself has many advantages over buying ready made meals. Importantly, you know what's in the food you're going to be eating, which given the recent horsemeat scandal, is not something that can be said for all foods. Home cooking also allows you to involve children in the process, making it a real family event, so it can help teach children about where food comes from and how it's made. In terms of weight management, home cooking allows you to cook exactly what you want, exactly how you want it. Some cooking techniques are healthier than others, some variations of the same type of food are healthier than others and some foods in the recipe can be swapped out for healthier ones. You have total control over what you cook, how you cook it and how you present it.

If your kitchen doesn't lend itself to cooking because equipment is hard to find, there's nowhere to prepare food or it's downright filthy, you're not going to cook. If you have an environment that makes it easy for you make your own food, you're going to appreciate the food more and understand food more than if you live off prepared and microwave meals.

Cooking meals yourself takes more time and it may not be practical to cook every night but if you increase the amount of food you cook at home and decrease the amounts of food from other sources, you give yourself an important way of successfully maintaining a healthy weight.

Fridge/Cupboards - when fancying a snack, the fridge and cupboard are the first places most people look. How you arrange them and what you choose to put in their in the first place. A good strategy involves placing anything unhealthy out of sight, whether it's at the back or covered in tin foil or baking paper or something. This is particularly true if the unhealthy foods belong to someone else in the house and not you, you don't want to be looking for some carrot sticks, realise someone put some leftover pizza in there and then go for that instead. You also want to make sure all the healthy food is right at the front and presented nicely so it's enticing and easy to grab. When you're starving or in a rush, you don't want to root around in the fridge trying to find good food, you want it right there, first thing you see.

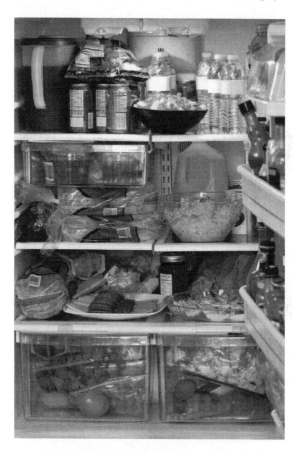

Countertop - again, it's all about what is in easy reach and in sight. Some house layouts require you to walk through the kitchen to get to other parts of the house such as a utility room, garage or garden. If you have to walk through the kitchen several times a day and you have unhealthy snacks easily available, there's a good chance you're going to eat them at some point. Salted peanuts, crisps, chocolates or biscuits are all foods that are commonly left out on the worktop for easy access. These also happen to be foods that can significantly add to your calorie intake. So have a clean countertop with the exception of some healthy snacks and a fruit bowl. A clean work top also means it's easier to freshly prepare and cook food as it means you don't have anything to do before you begin. Having to tidy up before you start can lead you to getting a ready meal or processed food out of the freezer rather than having fresh produce.

Work

The other place you are likely to spend a large portion of your time is your workplace. Everyone has different jobs and everyone has a different work space but most people will have some sort of desk in an office somewhere. The first thing you need to do is throw away or give away every bit of food that's in your snack drawer.

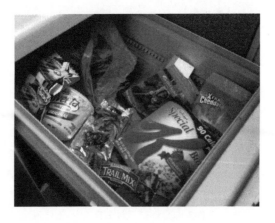

© Depositphotos.com/cdphotos

Most people's emergency stash for a late night or when they're tired consists of unhealthy food that is not going to help you lose any weight. You need to get rid of it and replace any emergency food with healthier options such as tinned fruit, a reasonable snack bar like a 9bar or a protein bar, some Ryvitas, rice cakes or oat cakes.

You also need to clear your desk of any chocolates or little bites that you may have available. It's common for nibbles like chocolates or crackers to be available at work for when you fancy one. If you don't fancy one, that's fine, but then in five minutes time, you glance at them again, look at your watch, see it's an hour until lunchtime and then have one. It's an impossible battle that you can't win. If there are some sweets within sight and reach of your desk and you glance at them every five minutes, you have to make the decision to not eat anything 12 times per hour, 96 mini decisions every working day. Only the very disciplined will win every battle. If they're out of sight, you may only think about them two or three times an hour. You're giving yourself chance to avoid eating these foods that you don't need. If every sweet is 50 calories and you have three per day, which seems too small and insignificant, you'll add 150 calories every day; which is 3,150 calories in a working month. I say 50 as an average, I am sure some types of sweet will be less and some will be more, I've known some chocolate truffles that contain 110 calories in a single marble sized chocolate.

If anyone brings in cakes, biscuits and other foods for a special occasion, try and move them to the other side of the office where you won't be constantly thinking about them. If you think you might succumb, have some fruit or some yoghurt or something to prevent yourself from reaching for anything once you are hungry. If someone offers you some cake for their birthday, have a look at the chapter "Would you not have a nice cup of tea?". Remember, you not eating food doesn't mean that you don't wish them happy birthday and you not having a glass of Buck's Fizz, doesn't mean you don't share in the celebration.

Having food in sight means you're more likely to eat it than if you have it out of sight, such as in a drawer. If you place the food in a drawer that's a short walk away or in another room, you're even less likely to dip into it.

Sometimes hunger can be mistaken for thirst and sometimes hunger is just you wanting to use your mouth to take in food or drink, like a comfort mechanism. If you have a 1 litre bottle of water on your desk in sight at all times you can have some water when you think you are hungry, then, wait 5 minutes or so and you may find the hunger sensation has disappeared.

Don't use a disposable bottle, buy a Nalgene bottle or something with measurements on so you can track your water intake. It's also handy to have on your desk and in sight so it reminds you of why it is there, this time it's OK to constantly keep having some!

Conclusion

None of these are big changes in themselves, but they

all add up to make a significant difference in the environments that you spend most time in, a difference that promotes activities that help you maintain a healthy weight. Why would you make things harder for yourself? You need to make having a healthy diet as easy as possible to obtain, don't give yourself unnecessary barriers or challenges, make sure your environment is as friendly and supportive as it can be.

Getting the right foundation in place to assist weight loss is going to really help you succeed. It does take effort and time and may take some getting used to, but your healthy weight won't automatically happen, you're going to make it happen!

The Nutritional Gatekeeper

I have some questions for you to think about.

• Who buys the food in your home?

• Who cooks the food in your home?

• What kind of food do they cook?

• What ingredients do they use?

• How much variety is there?

• Does that person buy / cook foods that you don't like?

• Does that person not buy things you do like?

• Do you wish they'd cook a particular dish you do like?

The reason I ask is because in 90% of cases, the person buying all the food in the home is the same person who cooks all the food in the home, which means that person has tremendous influence over what everyone eats. This person has been coined the Nutritional Gatekeeper, and is defined in a study by Brian Wansink, titled "Focus on Nutritional Gatekeepers", published in the Journal of the America Dietetic Association[1]. What this study found is that this person was responsible for 72% of the food related decisions for the people in their homes, i.e. their children and their spouse.

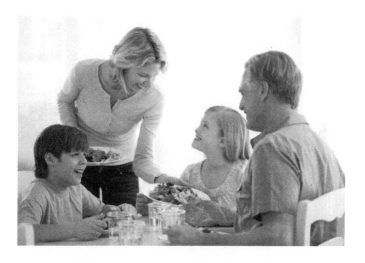

© Depositphotos.com/tmcphotos

As they are the chief shopper, they decide what to buy from the supermarket, what comes into the house and what food is available to the family. In fact, it's safe to say they define your very existence! Imagine your gatekeeper goes shopping when they're feeling in the mood for chocolate? By buying more chocolate, you open up the entire family to that same chocolate. What if they fancy some biscuits and they're on offer so they get two boxes. Those biscuits could very easily be yours.

There may be healthy versions of food that they don't buy because they pick the unhealthy version. For example, perhaps you ask for chips and they buy the American fries version, which uses much more oil than McCain oven chips.

As chief cook, they decide how to cook the food that they have bought. It may seem trivial but the method of cooking can make or break a meal from a weight loss perspective. Baking, steaming and roasting with a bit of oil are all good methods of cooking but perhaps your chief cook will fry, roast in lots of oil or add lots of butter to vegetables to make them taste better.

There may be healthy foods that you would benefit from eating but because the gatekeeper doesn't cook them properly or maybe they don't even buy them at all, you'll never have them as part of your diet.

If you want to change what you eat, you need the nutritional gatekeeper on board. You really have two options, the first is to make sure the gatekeeper is fully aware of your goal of losing weight and maintaining a healthy weight. They need to know exactly which food you like and exactly how you like it prepared.

The problem with this is that you give control away to the gatekeeper and you rely on them to do the work of shopping and cooking but also you let them make decisions that affect your goals. It also provides a convenient reason as to why you may not have achieved your goals and allows you to justify to yourself by blaming someone else. The second option is to not rely on the gatekeeper but to take control yourself. You shop for yourself and cook for yourself so that you control your food and drink. You could perhaps compromise, you could write a list of exactly what you require from the supermarket and let someone else shop for you so you get the ingredients you want and then you can still do the cooking yourself.

It might be that the gatekeeper is on board with your wish to change your diet so you can have be a healthy weight and they may decide that they want to be part of that, which is great news. Perhaps they already are a healthy weight and they just want to have a better diet, which means you now have some common interests. You may find the way to get their cooperation is by highlighting the benefits to your children of looking at what could be healthier in the weekly shop. Having them on board is easier than going it alone but there's still the possibility that they may not want change as much as you do. This gives you only one option, which is to take responsibility yourself.

Conclusion

If you choose to let the gatekeeper shop and cook for you and you do not meet your goal one week, no blame can be placed on the gatekeeper because you choose to give away your control to them and in giving away control you're also giving away your responsibility.

Chapter 4

How to Handle Your Hunger

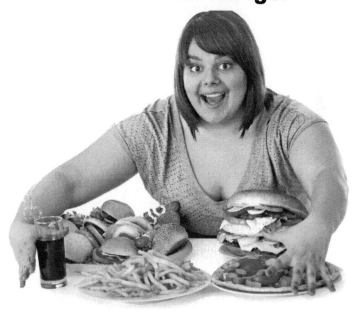

© Depositphotos.com/pozynakov

When I was learning German at school, there was a song in the textbook that we used to sing. It was a pretty simple song and it went like this: "Ich habe hunger hunger hunger, habe hunger hunger hunger, habe hunger hunger hunger, habe durst". It translates to "I have hunger, hunger, hunger , have hunger, hunger, hunger, have hunger hunger hunger, have thirst". Bet you could have worked that out, couldn't you?

I mention this because when feeling hungry, it's common to think about nothing else but how hungry you are. This pattern continues until you've managed to have some food. When I am coaching clients, I like to talk to them about hunger management and how we deal with hunger.

What is hunger? Hunger is defined as

1. a compelling need or desire for food.

2. the painful sensation or state of weakness caused by the need of food: to collapse from hunger.

When was the last time you said you were hungry? Was it number one or two of the definitions above? Or was it none of those? Most of us probably don't get to the second definition but how often do you hear yourself say "I'm starving", or, as I did when I was a child, "Mum, I'm starrrrrrrrrviiiiing!". Clearly I wasn't, but it was common for me to exaggerate my hunger level in order to get something to eat. I may have just wanted attention or was bored or it might have been for some other reason, but the majority of the time I wasn't really that hungry. Over a number of years my hunger detection was distorted so even a slight hunger got ramped up to starving.

Hunger is a very important aspect of weight management and is often confused for something else. The table below shows the differences between hunger and things that aren't hunger.

Hunger	Something else
Builds gradually	Comes on suddenly
Is felt below the neck (e.g. stomach rumbling)	Is felt above the neck (e.g. craving for chocolate)
Occurs several hours after a meal	Occurs any time
Goes away when full	Can occur when full
Eating leads to feeling of satisfaction	Eating leads to guilt and shame

The things that aren't hunger can not be satisfied by eating. This makes sense, doesn't it? If whatever you feel isn't hunger, food is not the answer to it.

Can you think of other things that may be mistaken for hunger? Here are a few common ones:

· Boredom

· Anxiousness

· Excitement

· Worry

· Sadness

- Guilt

- Fear

- Joy

- Shame

- Nervousness

- Mental tiredness

This is not an exhaustive list, but does highlight just how many different things can be interpreted as hunger. The problem this presents us with is that if we interpret things as hunger that aren't hunger, we may eat a lot more than we need to. I just want to clarify again, if you are feeling any of the above then food or drink will not help you one bit.

So this chapter will focus on hunger, when to eat and when to stop eating.

Hunger

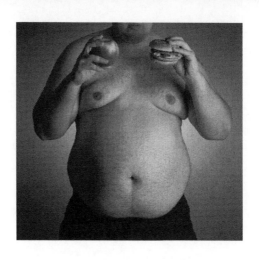

The first step in mastering the habits of hunger is to identify the different types of hunger, as written by Jan Chozen Bays, a paediatrician and Zen teacher from Oregon in America. She defines seven types of hunger, which are stomach hunger, cellular hunger, nose hunger, heart hunger, eye hunger, mind hunger as mouth hunger.

This is an interesting concept as it does highlight just how many signals you can receive from your body and what a job you have to correctly interpret them.

Stomach hunger – I think most of us are familiar with this one. We've all had a growling or rumbling stomach but the stomach doesn't control us, we control the stomach. The stomach becomes conditioned to expect food at particular times, so when you go on holiday, the stomach can adjust accordingly with our wishes. Have you ever had a stomach rumble but not been able to do anything about it, and then the stomach rumbling has gone away? This could be because it wasn't really hunger in the first place, it could be anxiety, heartburn, indigestion or other feelings. So it would be best to wait a little while before eating rather than have a meal the minute you feel a rumble.

Cellular hunger – this is the craving side of hunger. We have to eat because the cells of our bodies are craving some nutrient or other. Sometimes we think our cells are craving something but actually it's simply thirst. So when you think you're craving, try and have a drink first. Also, think about what you might be craving, for the reason you are craving it is because your body needs it. If you are craving fast food, it is unlikely that this is because of cellular hunger as usually you will crave nutrients rather than junk food.

Nose hunger – have you ever been in a house when someone is baking buns and the minute you sense the smell, you become hungry? Or you got a whiff of a smell that took you back to your childhood and suddenly felt like you must have that particular food again? So if the hunger is prompted by the smell, could you do without it?

Heart hunger – maybe experiencing smell of someone baking buns or cakes or whatever brings back memories of when you were a child and suddenly makes you want a jam tart. When you eat it, you can relive that moment and experience those feelings again. This would be one of the things that would satisfy heart hunger. Another example is using food to take away emotional upset or anxiety, which is very common for people to do.

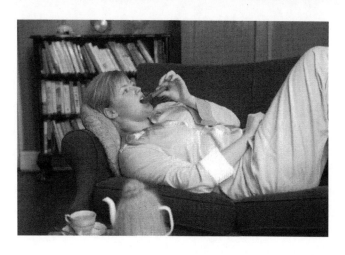

Eye hunger – Eye hunger is where your eyes are bigger than your stomach. Have you ever finished a meal and been stuffed full of food and unable to eat anything more? Then you see the dessert trolley and suddenly you must have the cake, the crumble and the ice cream? You've become hungry because your eyes have become larger than your stomach. If you find yourself in this position, try looking at something else that you find pretty and attractive so your eyes can get their fix.

Mind hunger – this is when your mind is telling you what you should and shouldn't eat. Perhaps you've had a long day and deserve an ice cream or have been to the gym so deserve a pizza. Maybe you have one more potato on your plate, you feel full but your mind says that you could manage just one more. The inner voice can also work the other way and tell you what you shouldn't have so it's important to make sure you don't follow the orders without questioning.

Mouth hunger – this is where your mouth drives your need for food. You want to feel the sensation of eating or chewing. The mouth wants a particular sensation or taste, so it is important to chew your food as many times as you can so that you don't over consume.

One of the most important things I tell my clients is how to recognise genuine hunger and distinguish it from all the other signals we get. If I ate every time I thought I was hungry, I'd probably eat twice as often as I do now.

How to achieve correct recognition of hunger is a genuine skill and it takes time, almost like trying to differentiate between different bird songs, you won't be able to identify signals straight away but over time you are able to filter out the spurious signals and tune in to what your body is actually telling you.

Mindful Moments - When to Eat

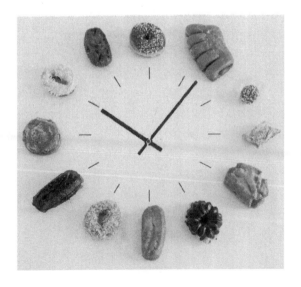

71

One really good strategy to avoid eating when you're not really hungry is to take a mindful moment before you eat. A Mindful Moment is you checking with yourself and asking yourself what's happening. To get the information, you need to ask yourself some questions.

When you start to feel some sort of hunger, work through these questions below and see what answers you receive.

1. Which type of hunger is this, which bit of my body is the signal coming from?

2. What do I hope to achieve by eating this?

3. Are there any drawbacks to this?

4. Could I replace food with something else to achieve the same thing?

For example, if you were about to go to the kitchen for a bar of chocolate, you could give yourself a Mindful Moment before going into the kitchen and you could answer the questions above, perhaps as this example:

1. It's probably heart hunger because I am bored.

2. Pass the time.

3. I might be bored again after eating it and I'll feel guilty or I'll continue eating.

4. I could go for a walk and get some fresh air.

In that Mindful Moment, that person had enough time to THINK about what they were about to do, ask WHY they were doing it and worked out it was not the right solution for that situation.

Mindful Moments take literally two minutes and unless you are on the verge of collapsing, I think you should be able to wait a couple of minutes before you eat. It's well worth taking the time to do this little exercise, even if it feels unusual at first. If your car was making funny noises and maybe not performing as usual, you wouldn't just automatically respond to whatever the issue was by providing it more fuel. It might need a water top up, the cam belt changing or some air in the tyres. Your body operates in a similar way, by giving off signals it is alerting you to an issue and you need to take time to investigate what those signals mean before deciding on the response. Responding with food when hunger isn't the issue is a guaranteed way to eat more than necessary.

It's important to note that if you are not eating because of genuine hunger, eating will not satisfy you. If you are in tune with your body enough to realise it's not hunger, here are some ideas for what could help be an alternative action than eating. How often have you eaten just because you were bored? I used to stand in front of the fridge or cupboard longingly staring inside for some magical food to pop out so I could eat it. I wasn't really hungry, I was bored. Looking for food and then eating it gave me a nice distraction from being bored.

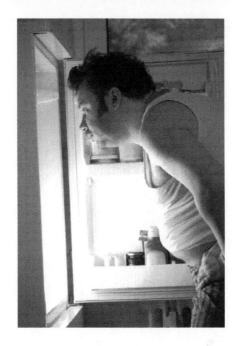

Having a distraction or giving yourself a non-food reward can usually remove the feelings that masqueraded as hunger. A few ideas are below:

• Walk to the shops and buy your favourite magazine

• Buy yourself a bunch of flowers

• Paint nails or toenails (possibly women only)

• Go to the cinema

• Tweet something

• Buy a £3 DVD (maybe not from the supermarket) and have a film night

- Ring a friend and have a laugh

- Watch a funny Youtube video for 5 minutes

- Shop for a cheap treat or buy someone a present

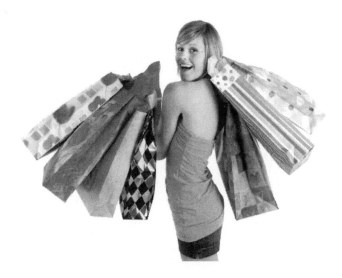

© Depositphotos.com/cybernesco

- Watch favourite recorded TV programme

- Internet browsing for fun

- Write a card to a loved one and tell them something nice

- Have a long bath with scented bubble bath

- Listen to some music while taking a walk round the block

- Browse through a photo album and relive some happy

memories

- Read a chapter of the book you are currently reading

- Buy a comic strip book, e.g. Dilbert, Garfield, Calvin & Hobbes etc. and read a few

- Put on a CD, sit down and relax and close your eyes whilst listening to the music

- Plan your weekend, write down what you're going to do

- Tweet/Facebook something. Find someone new to follow or add a new friend.

When to Stop Eating

When do you stop eating? Think about it, you have food in front of you, you have begun eating whatever food it is, but at what point do you stop? How do you know when to stop eating?

A study was done by Cornell University, in which participants were invited to a restaurant and served soup in soup bowls. The soup bowls were specially crafted so they refilled constantly and the amount of soup in it never went down. There were vats of soup under the table that were connected by tube to the soup bowls to prevent the bowl running out of soup. The soup bowls were bottomless, so they never emptied and therefore the participants of the study could not rely on an empty bowl to work out when to finish. Half of the people in the study had a bottomless bowl and half had a normal bowl.

The people eating from the bottomless bowls ate 73% more than those with normal bowls, but they did not feel they had eaten more. This shows just how much we rely on external cues to guide our eating and our perception about how much we have eaten.

Another study involved dividing a bar into two halves, and having a waitress service for each. The bar was serving a special on chicken wings that night. The waitresses on one half of the bar were told to clear away the chicken wing bones from the tables but the waitresses on the other half of the bar were told to leave them on the table. The people sitting at tables where the bones remained behind ate 28% less than the people who had no indication of how much that had eaten because the bones had been cleared away.

Most people use external cues to know when to stop eating, common ones are:

• When my plate is empty

• When I've read the paper

• When the television programme has finished

Compare these to your answers. None of these are related to your body or the needs of your body. They are all external cues and allow your decisions to be influenced by external factors, taking the control away from you about when you should stop eating. If you rely on external cues, you are giving away control and not doing what your body wants or needs. This can lead to overeating.

I'll talk more about strategies for managing your individual meal intake later in Successful Portion Control, but I want to highlight the skill of identifying at what point you need to stop eating.

When we are children, it's common for our parents to ask us "Are you full yet?" when we're eating. When I was a child I would answer "No" and my parents would make sure I had more to eat. One consequence of questions like this is that it conditions you to stop eating when you're full. I believe that we should stop eating when we are no longer hungry. To highlight the difference, have a look at the satiety scale below. The Mindful Moment can also be useful here. You can use it mid meal to assess your satiety. As you can see from the scale, there's a big difference between no longer being hungry and either being totally full or being in pain due to eating too much. There is also a big difference in calories, stopping eating when you're no longer hungry can save you a lot of calories than if you stop eating when you can physically eat no more.

10	You feel very uncomfortable, perhaps somewhat painful and you may be sick.	*You have over eaten and the signals your body has given off have not been listened to. You need to identify the reasons for this to prevent it happening again.*
9	You are starting to feel uncomfortable because you have eaten so much.	
8	You are not feeling uncomfortable, but full, with no more food wanted.	*Stop eating and let your body digest what you have eaten.*
7	You are comfortably satisfied and have no more hunger. You could go without food for 3 more hours.	*This is a good place to stop as moving to level 8 hunger will not satisfy you more but will increase your calorie intake. If you are not hungry there is no reason to continue to eat.*
6	You could eat more but are no longer hungry.	
5	You are not hungry and not full. You have no strong feelings either way.	*If you are likely to be hungry in the near future, it may be worth thinking about having food available so you don't get to level 2 hunger.*
4	A little hungry. You could wait some time before eating but you know you will be more hungry as time progresses.	

3	You are hungry and need to eat.	*Take the time to prepare something to eat so that you can satisfy the hunger sensation.*
2	You are aware of physical sensation of hunger and it is preoccupying you. You may eat things that you would not normally eat.	*This is a time to be aware that your extreme hunger could lead you to making poor food choices. Listen to your body and make a note of the signals given off so that you can avoid level 1 and 2 stage hunger.*
1	Your are almost in pain with your hunger and you will eat anything.	

You want to avoid extremes of hunger and satiety. Being level one or two hunger increases the chances that you'll reach for something unhealthy just to satisfy your want of food. Reach level nine or ten hunger means you've eaten more than your body wanted and have taken in unnecessary calories.

Conclusion

- The Mindful Moment employed before eating can help you assess where you are the scale, whether it's a three and eating might be a good idea or whether it's a five and actually you could quite happily last another hour or two without any food. Using the Mindful Moment mid meal allows you to prevent reaching the nine or ten levels and allows you to be aware of your body enough to stop at either six, seven or eight.

- Assessing whether you are really hungry or not, working out when to eat and working out when to stop eating are important skills to practice if you want to lose weight or maintain a healthy weight.

- Be honest when you're asking yourself about how hungry you are and what you think the real reason for the feeling is, then you'll be better placed to take the right course of action. It will not be hunger every time.

Chapter 5

Gone in 60 Seconds

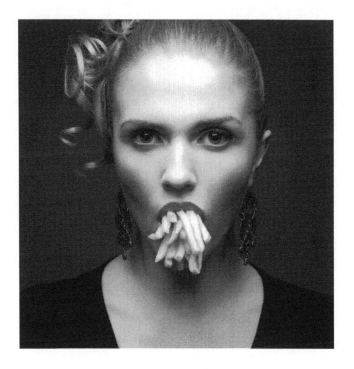

© Depositphotos.com/avgustino

Do you remember the Flake adverts of the 70s and 80s? With the woman in the bath and the sexy music and the steam rising from the water? Do you remember how she ate the Flake and just enjoyed the moment? The slogan was "Cadbury's Flake, the crumbliest, most flakiest chocolate in the world". Say what you want about that advert but she was enjoying that Flake, and the nation was enjoying watching her.

Compare that to the way our pet dog Scamp, used to eat his dinner. I'm sure all pet owners out there can relate to pet feeding time. He would have his mouth in the bowl before I'f finished putting the food in, and then he would not look up until he'd finished. His bowl used to move around the room like it had a mind of its own as he gobbled down the food in about 60 seconds.

Have you ever driven home from work and not been able to remember anything about your commute? You drove home on autopilot because you do that route so often you don't really need to concentrate and you can think about something else, such as what you're going to do at the weekend or how the project at work is coming along.

The Flake woman was paying attention to her Flake. She didn't care that the bath was overflowing or that she might be exposing a bit too much of herself, she just wanted to enjoy the moment with her Flake.

All that Scamp wanted was to wolf down his dinner as quickly as possible, and it's surprising how quickly a Westie can do that!

When you're driving home all you want is to be home and you want the commute to be over.

Scamp had an excuse; he was a dog, you are not a dog. Therefore there should be some important differences between the way you eat and the way Scamp, bless him, used to eat. The Flake woman had the right idea by making it an experience and enjoying it. The key to her success was mindfulness.

Mindfulness is an important aspect of a healthy relationship with food. You may have heard of a method of eating called Mindful Eating or perhaps, Mindless Eating, which is what many of us do. Mindful Eating can be defined as:

Being aware of how your body is feeling, i.e. are you hungry, it means eating food without judgement or emotion, being aware of what is happening, paying attention, savouring the process of eating and the food or drink being consumed and being aware of when you are no longer hungry.

Knowing when you are hungry is discussed in the chapter on hunger.

Eating without judgement means not thinking that the food you are eating is bad or good, it means eating the food without any negative thoughts.

Being aware of what is happening is really important, being free of distractions and focussing on your meal will really help you experience a sense of satisfaction from your meal.

Mindfulness is a brilliant and superbly useful technique than make a big difference to your life but to get the benefits, you need to use it. To help you understand how it can be used, I want you to think about some things that you do that might be fun. Here are some examples below:

- Spending time with your child

- A ride in a fast sports car

- A balloon ride over the countryside

- An expensive meal

- Your favourite television programme

- Wildlife watching

- Watching your favourite team win a big game

- Meeting your idol

- A first date with that special someone

- Reading a good book

- Celebrating scoring the winning goal

Add your own to the list if these aren't applicable to you. Think about how you might experience them. They are special, you enjoy them and you want to make the most of them.

I will give my own example, from a holiday in Alaska. I was sat on a rock in the middle of nowhere and about a couple of miles away was a mile wide, 6 mile long glacier called Meares Glacier. There were only five of us there and the sky was clear with the sun shining on us. Every so often the glacier would calve and we would see the ice fall into the sea and two seconds later, we'd hear it as the sound travelled the two miles to us. We sat there most of the day, just enjoying the weather, the wildlife and the glacier. I can still recall the scene even now; I was sat there and I closed my eyes for a few seconds to reset myself, concentrating just on the sounds, then I would open my eyes to see the splendour of the scene that I was lucky enough to be a part of. I did this several times so I could get all aspects of the scene into my memory because I knew I might never go back. I'm on the left in the photo below.

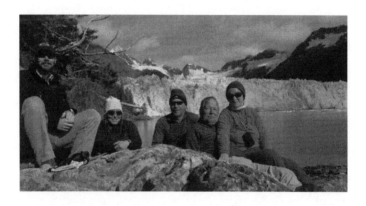

I could have approached that differently, I could have let my mind wander to what might be happening at home, I could have closed my eyes and sunbathed or I could have listened to music on my MP3 player and relaxed that day. But I didn't. I made sure every single one of my senses was tuned in to that scene so that I could get the maximum from it.

Think about when you eat, where is your attention? Where are your senses directed? What else are you doing besides eating? Do you get everything you can from the food experience? Even reading this book, is your mind reading and taking in the words or are you just glossing over it thinking about something else? It's common for us to allow ourselves to be distracted because we have such busy lives and there are so many things going on.

Would your driving be better if you focussed on it? Would you get the most out of a book because you're fully concentrating on it? Would you learn more in your language class if you gave it your full attention? The answer to all those is absolutely, so let's give our current task priority and give it the focus and direct attention it deserves.

Being mindful will help you maximise the benefits or effectiveness from whatever you're doing. I'm going to concentrate on eating, given the content of this book.

When you eat or drink, you want to try and gain maximum satisfaction, let all your senses be in tune with whatever it is you are about to eat or drink; it's not just about satisfying your taste buds. I'll give you an example. Consider you are in a nice restaurant. The decor is nice, your cutlery is clean, the place setting is ready and the company is good. You're looking forward to your chosen dish of cheese and spinach ravioli with a thick mushroom sauce and a side order of roasted vegetables.

You're already looking forward to the food and your body is tuned in for the nice meal that is on its way, this gets your mind ready for eating. The waiter brings it to the table, places it gently in front of you and then leaves you to begin your meal. This is where your eyes get satisfaction from looking at the food and your sense of smell kicks in as you enjoy the smell and your body begins to prepare itself for food. Then you feel the food with the knife and fork, cutting into the ravioli, feeling the soft pasta split and the filling oozing out, providing you with a new texture and new smell.

You load it onto your fork and slowly bring it towards your mouth. You open your mouth, let your tongue taste the ravioli, maybe closing your eyes to really immerse yourself in the moment as you let your tongue taste the ravioli. As you begin to chew more, you taste more of the filling, continuing to chew to really taste the whole bite, then you swallow that bite and open your eyes ready for the next.

Now, I'm not saying you need to hit ecstasy every time you eat but what I am saying is that you need to value the food and savour it, otherwise you might as well just live off the blandest, cheapest food you can buy and take supplements to get your nutritional needs met.

If you consistently eat on autopilot, you run the risk of overeating. If you are tuned in and in control when you are eating, you can reduce the risk of over eating. In the example, our mind was satisfied because we were looking forward to the food, our eyes were satisfied because we took time to look at the food before getting started, our smell was satisfied because we could smell the food on the table but also when we bring it to our mouths to eat and our taste buds were satisfied because we took time to taste the food. Our ears weren't satisfied with ravioli but it could have been the sound of a crisp Yorkshire Pudding cracking or the packaging of a chocolate bar being open. An important concept to remember is food is not just about taste, it's about your whole body, after all, the nourishment you are taking in is used by your entire body.

Let me give you a simple equation:

$$\text{Total Satisfaction} = \frac{\text{Satisfaction per Bite}}{\text{Number of Bites}}$$

So one of our mindful eating aims is to get the most pleasure, enjoyment and satisfaction that is available from each meal. Eating can be an enjoyable experience, so why would we not want to get the most from it? If it's not satisfying, why are we eating it? If we don't feel satisfied when we've eaten, it's likely that we'll eat more that we need to, which is not good as a weight management strategy.

Here are a few practical ways in which you can change the way you eat to get maximum satisfaction from what you're eating.

- Give yourself 30 seconds before you start eating to just look at the meal and enjoy the presentation of the food. If you are preparing the food yourself, take time to do this, if it looks rubbish, there's less chance you'll find satisfaction as you will have already started on a negative. Presentation is important, it sets the meal up to be nice; there's a good reason why restaurants take care with their presentation. Notice the colours, shapes and arrangements on the plate.

- Load small bite sized portions onto the fork and chew at least 30 times, preferably 40 times. This sounds like a lot, but it really isn't. I recently watched someone eat a carvery and they had the biggest chunk of meat and just golloped it down in two bites. Two bites! How can you taste that? He probably only tasted the gravy. Food is meant to be chewed, this means you can taste more, when you taste more, you eat less. If you swallow it whole you're not tasting anything, most of the surface area of the food is still as it was on the plate, meaning you've missed out on most of the taste. You fancy a bit more of that so you have more food. You've actually had enough food but have eaten it in such an inefficient way that you require much more to get the same taste satisfaction. Chewing also allows your body to digest it more effectively. Carbohydrate digestion begins in the mouth and for meats you need to chew to allow digestion to work effectively in the stomach. Having large chunks of undigested food moving through your digestive system can give you problems and prevents nutrients from being extracted and absorbed into your body. Chewing is really important, more taste means more satisfaction.

- Don't load up the next forkful until you've swallowed what you had on the last forkful. It's not a race and you're supposed to be enjoying the taste of the food in your mouth. If the taste is not worth concentrating on, why are you so keen for another mouthful?

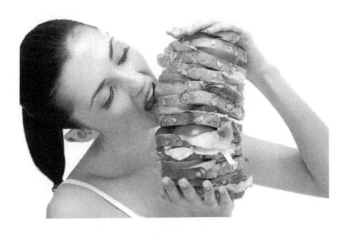

© Depositphotos.com/luckybusiness

- Put the knife and fork down whilst you're chewing if this helps you. You'll slow your meal down this way and it will give you time to talk to the people that you are with. The digestive system in your body is incredibly complex and able, but it takes 20 minutes for the necessary hormones in your digestive system to reach your brain. These are the hormones that indicate satiety or hunger so your brain can respond accordingly, there are sensors in your stomach that detect when the stomach is full and the slower you eat, the more time you give your body to register what is happening. If you wolf your food down in 10 minutes, your body has no time to respond to tell you that you aren't hungry any more. By the time you get that signal you're way past no longer hungry and into an uncomfortable feeling and your calorie intake has gone up.

- Pace yourself with the slowest eater at the table, this will help you set a rhythm and establish a change in your normal behaviour. Surely you want the meal experience to last longer without having more food?

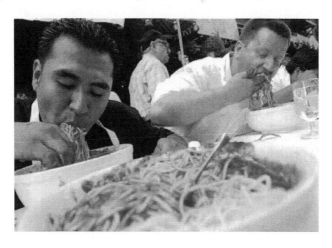

- Sit down and eat your meal at the table, with a place setting. This means you have a good posture, you're not slouched on settee somewhere and half heartedly putting the effort in. Every meal might not need to be like this but certainly the evening meal should be.

- Try and make the meal last for at least 20 minutes. This can be achieved by the ideas above but you could set a timer on your phone, just to give you an idea of how long it takes now and then you know how much longer you should take. It's also a very satisfying feeling when you eat with others and they've polished all theirs off and you're still got some of the lovely food left on your plate to enjoy.

- If you're with other people and are enjoying talking during the meal, don't rush a mouthful just to fill the gap in conversation. I often see people take a bite and quickly swallow because they have something they want to say. It's a waste of a bite, so concentrate on chewing and tasting rather than getting it down you so quickly just so you can carry on talking.

I know it's not practical for every time you eat to be the special occasion and sensory treat for your taste buds that makes a mindful meal as satisfying as can be. I'm well aware of the practicalities of life but I am also well aware you might be trying to either lose weight of more effectively manage your weight. The ideas I've talked about here make a difference, even if it's just once a day for your evening meal. It's your responsibility then to try and introduce the habits into other meals.

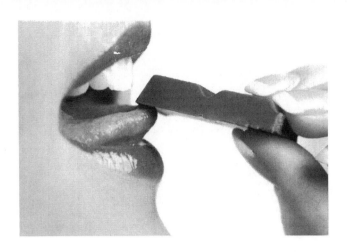

A good example is chocolate, lots of people like chocolate and it's a particular must have for many people. If you're going to eat chocolate, which is a high fat and high sugar food, eating it mindfully is the other way to do it. It's common for people to eat an unhealthy food as quickly as they can to get the guilt over and done with. Eating mindfully means eating without guilt and maximum enjoyment from the food. It's often said that the first two bites of dessert are the best because you gain maximum pleasure from these bites because they are new, after that it becomes a bit samey and you're just eating it to finish off the portion. If you eat mindfully, you'll find you need less of the foods like chocolate because you'll get all the enjoyment and pleasure from a smaller amount of food.

Conclusion

- I want you to try approaching things a bit more mindfully, focussing on the food and not distracting yourself with something else. Food is important and deserves to be given your attention.

- Compare the difference in experience between eating something mindfully and eating something without really thinking about it. See if the benefits highlight themselves to you, identify the differences between each way of eating.

- Try and put distractions aside, leave the phone, laptop, tablet, newspaper somewhere else and turn off the television. Focus on the food.

Chapter 6

Behaviour for Successful Weight Loss

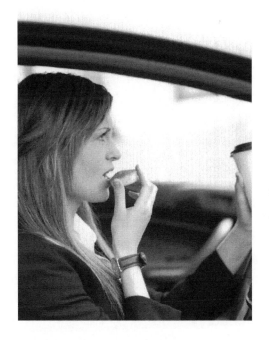

© Depositphotos.com/Wavebreakmedia

Established Habits

When I was a child, during my school years, my Mum would walk to the school gate and collect us so we could all walk home together. Without fail, every time my brother and I walked in from school, there would be some sweets for us, always in the same place on the kitchen side, my brother's on one side and mine on the other. A packet of Maltesers, a Milky Way or behold, the holy grail of after school sweets, some Mini Eggs.

This progressed into my adult and working life (no, not having sweets waiting for when I got home), but the association I built between arriving home and eating. I couldn't help it, I would always feel the need to eat when I came in from somewhere. It didn't matter whether it was a night out or if I was coming home from work and tea was going to be ready in the next half hour, I always felt the need to eat. My usual choice was a bowl of cereal and I'm convinced this need to eat that bore no relation to how hungry I was, how much I'd eaten that day or anything else, is because of the repeated eating when coming home from school that became an established habit over a number of years.

Have you ever been really busy in the morning, and the day has just flown by and you wonder what time it is? You see it's 11:45 or maybe 12:00 or something like that and suddenly you feel hungry. There was no hunger before but because you've now seen it's approaching lunch time or is past lunch time, you're starving and need to eat.

A great example of established habits is the cinema. If you have been to the cinema recently you'll notice that before you go in to the cinema you can buy something to drink and you can buy something to eat. You can buy food and drink that come in colossal containers. You have the soft drinks, popcorn, bags of sweets, sticky lollies and the pick and mix. Then, either before or during the film, someone thinks that isn't quite enough and offers you some ice cream to keep you going. With the exceptions of Lord of the Rings and Titanic, most films at the cinema are about an hour and a half and yet we bring in with us food with enough calories to last us over a day.

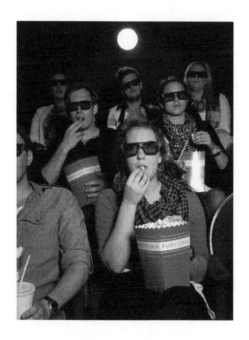

© Depositphotos.com/genenacom

We do this because these are habits that are entrenched within us. The associations we have build up over our lives, whether by the culture of our society or something specific with your upbringing, everyone has their own habits that are established and become their norms.

There are accepted norms within society or within our family that dictate to us what we should eat, how much we should eat and when we should eat. I'm going to give some common examples, some may apply to you and some may not, but I guarantee that you'll have been influenced by at least one of them.

- You eat breakfast until you've read the paper, even if it means refilling your bowl or place until the paper has been read

- It's a special occasion so we'll have some cake to celebrate

- We're going on a flight so we'll have some nuts

- You always eat breakfast on the go because you have no time to sit down properly

- Watching a sporting event so we'll have crisps, crackers and dips

- Eat all the food on my place, everyone else is still eating so have seconds until they are done

- It's lunch hour at work, let's walk to the shops

- Today is Takeaway Tuesday or Fish and Chip Friday

- I'll have a morning paper from the shop and I'll also take my morning Yorkie bar

- We're going round to visit our friends, let's take some biscuits and chocolates with us

- It's Christmas so we'll have nuts and chocolates about the house and on the tree

- I'm in a restaurant so I'll have some bread before my meal

- It's Friday night, hard week of work, I need 5 pints

There are lots of example of customs and habits that we all have in certain situations, repeated ways in which we behave that mean we eat certain foods or drink certain drinks. Can you think of any examples that are specific to you? There are many situations where the way we behave is driven by the social norm, almost etiquette, if you like.

Eating Out

Do you eat differently when you eat out? Think about how eating out is different from when you eat in?

Here are a few examples of how it can be different:

- Bread and butter/oil or olives to start

- A glass of wine before your meal

- Your meal might be three courses

- Coffee and mints to finish

- Feels like an occasion so time for treats

When eating out, there is a lot of opportunity for eating more than you need. The restaurant may have a different way of doing things to you. How often, at home, would you have bread before your starter? Or even have a starter? What about dessert? Food comes a lot easier as well, if you want more, you just have to ask and you'll get what you want without having to leave your seat. Eating out provides lots of opportunities for you to eat more than you need.

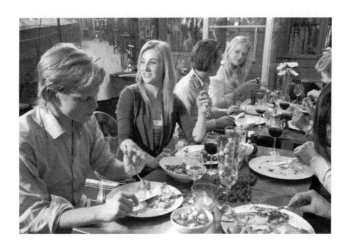

© Depositphotos.com/Corepics

To deal with this issue, decide how much you want as you sit down. This is where you have your Mindful Moment and ask yourself how hungry you are. To get you in the mood for more food and to keep everyone happy by giving them something to nibble, you're served bread at a restaurant. It may be beautifully smelling freshly baked bread that makes your nose inhale with delight (nose hunger) or it may be a golden brown squishy soft fluffy bread that has a wonderful texture and you fancy a taste (eye and mouth hunger) but it could also be the leftovers from other tables, which, if you knew, might not be so appetising! So you're sat there, other people are eating their meals, everyone on your table is eating bread, it's natural for you to want to eat bread. Sometimes it's served with butter or olive oil, but even on it's own it can be quite calorific.

Rather than consume these empty calories and fill up on bread rather than the good food you've come here for (Tripadvisor rarely features reviews of the bread), push the bread away to the other side of the table and make sure you have a glass of water if you need to eat or drink something.

Three's Company

Have you ever noticed anything different about your intake when you are with different people? Or when you are with more people? For example, when you go round to someone's house as a guest you might not ask for seconds whereas when your mum's doing a Sunday roast, you'll finish everything available.

Professor John DeCastro conducted a study to ascertain how much we eat when we have company and how this compares to when we eat alone[1]. He found that if you eat with one person, you'll eat 35% more than you would have eaten if you were alone. The percentage increases as the number of people you eat with increases. Eating with three other people gives you a 75% rise and eating with six or more people nearly doubles your intake as you eat 96% more.

You may not believe these figures but if you think about it, it's quite realistic. How many times do you have a starter or dessert because someone else is having one? Or you might share a starter together even though you weren't really bothered? You may not even have a starter, but you'll polish off the bread and oil before your main course because you can't watch someone else eat without eating yourself. You could share a side order or finish off the chips that they didn't want.

These are all way to take on unnecessary calories and it is important you are aware of how your behaviour can be influenced by your environment when eating out.

Eating In

Our habits most greatly influence us when we are at home, as this is where many of us eat breakfasts and our evening meals. This is the area that you control, you own and the changes you can make in this area have a really big effect.

• Do you always have the same breakfast?

• Have you ever tried making it healthier in any way?

- Do you always eat lunch at the same time?

- Is your lunch generally the same thing?

- Are your snacks always the same?

- Do you always have a dessert with your lunch?

- Are your drinks pretty much the same each day?

- Do you eat with your food on your lap watching the TV?

- Do you eat whilst reading the paper?

The most beneficial single change you can make to your evening meal habit is to eat at the table. I mentioned this briefly in the chapter on mindfulness but it really is an important aspect of weight management. This is partly due to the side benefits this brings such as making the meal more of an experience with a set table, it encourages conversation to make the meal last longer, it gives you better posture helping digestion, it encourages better table etiquette making the food last longer and it allows you to eat without distraction. There is one other key aspect of eating at the table; it stops you from eating in front of the television.

Bellyvision

Alaska is going to get a second mention here because there is a bar in Anchorage that I'd like to tell you about. It's a sports bar and it's called The Peanut Farm. I have watched a few sporting events there and enjoy it very much. When I first went, though, I had a bit of a culture shock because I'd never seen such a place. They have 70 television screens, some on the wall, some at the end of the tables and some above the bar. Here's a picture to help you visualise.

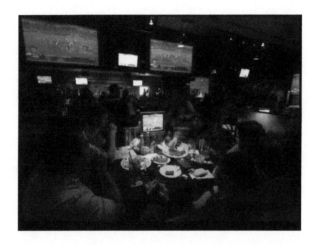

I can't help but laugh when I look at the family in this picture, all of them staring at the screen and all of them totally immersed in what they're watching. Sadly for them, they are all oblivious to the amount of deep fried food that they are quickly shovelling into their mouths. This is the ultimate example of how television can totally render you unconscious to your eating actions.

This may be a sports bar and perhaps this is not going to be such a regular thing for a family that it won't really make much difference but it isn't just sports bars that can hypnotise you while you eat.

How often do you watch television whilst eating? How often do you sit in front of the computer whilst eating? How often do you use your phone or tablet computer whilst eating? Whether it's a sports bar, your home or work, eating whilst you are fixated on something else isn't a good idea if you want to make sure you don't overeat. 60% of people eat their meals in front of the television so it occurs frequently enough that it would be useful to change our behaviour so this wasn't the dominant method of eating[2].

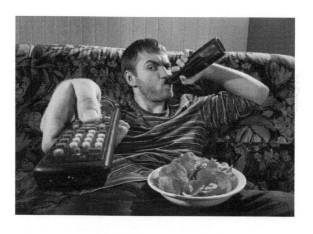

© Depositphotos.com/nomadsoul1

People in the UK watch on average four hours television each day. The fact so many people are eating in front of the television suggests that either the programmes are brilliant (Arrange Me a Marriage, Paris Hilton's New British Best Friend and I Shot My Face Off don't exactly scream brilliance to me) or people are doing what they've always done, driven by their established habits. We watch, on average, four hours of television a day[5]. Add that up over a year and it's two months a year sat watching TV. Thankfully, I don't watch that much television, but if I was reading this, and I just realised I spend two months of my year sat watching television, I would be pretty shocked right now.

Television contributes to over eating in several ways. Television can induce eating in the first place because of an established habit, such as watching a film and having some nibbles and fizzy drinks. Television can keep you eating for longer because the programme you are watching hasn't finished, you think that you might as well get a bit more food to keep you going until the end. I used to suffer from this one particularly, as well eating as I was reading the paper. I would always have a second bowl of cereal until the paper was read or the programme was nearly finished. My second bowl of cereal meant I'd eat 100% more but when you're in front of the television you eat between 31% and 74% more food. That's a lot of extra calories.

Advert breaks are a terrible thing in terms of weight loss. 15% of all adverts on television are food related and about 51% of those are to do with unhealthy or fast foods. Research shows that people will eat more food when they have been exposed to television adverts relating to food[3]. The type of food, whether it is a fun food, a healthy food or an unhealthy food can have an influence on what type of food is eaten. Children were found to eat 45% more food when exposed to television advertising[4].

The other thing advert breaks do is give you an opportunity to go and do something with your time, such as make a cup of coffee and have a biscuit. The National Grid say the most common surges are associated with television events and advert breaks. After the Coronation Street tram disaster of 2010, 300,000 people switched on their kettles afterwards[6], and perhaps not all had something to eat, but I am sure some of them had an unnecessary biscuit or cake to go with their drink.

Television is the number one enemy of mindful eating. How many times do you eat food that you rarely look at because your eyes are fixated on the television or computer screen? You might as well be eating prison food if you're not even going to pay attention to it.

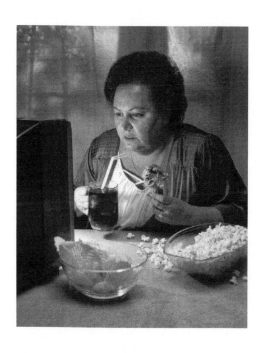

There is a risk that you end up not registering what you've eaten due to your lack of attention and then have something else after you've finished watching TV. This is because you didn't get any satisfaction from your meal. With the prevalence of catch up television online and hard disk recorders, you can put off the television until after you've eaten and you don't have to sit through the adverts, either. We've already talked about how beneficial it is to sit at the table for a meal, which has multiple benefits, not least keeping you away from the television.

If you can introduce this into your routine, you may find it has other benefits for you. If you're eating alone, I realise you might be a bit lonely, but you can still enjoy some relaxation time to enjoy your meal. Some time out from your day can reduce stress, which can lead to weight gain.

If you are eating with your partner, wouldn't you prefer to talk about how you day has been and what you'll be doing at the weekend and spend some quality time with them rather than sit in silence staring at the television?

If you are eating with your children, eating at the table introduces good habits as well as being linked with lower cases of obesity. This also serves as quality time together and gives you an opportunity to establish routines with your children. Some dietary habits are established in childhood so it's important to establish habits that promote a good diet rather than habits that promote a poor diet. If your children regularly eat their meals at the table with you, they will have a greater intake of fruit and vegetables than children who never eat at the table.

I appreciate and understand it may not be practical to eat every meal at the table but I would ask you to challenge yourself if you don't think you can achieve this at least three times a week. I think you'll find the five minutes it takes to prepare the table mean you will enjoy the experience more as you can eat mindfully, enjoy some conversation and jokes with your friends or family and avoid distractions that prevent you from the trap of sitting in front of a screen transferring food from plate to mouth in a mindless and robotic way.

Lost Lunches

How many times have you eaten your lunch at work whilst you are:

• Working at your desk

• Reading emails on your computer

• In a meeting

• Walking from the shops back to work

• Talking to someone else about work in your office

• Driving?!

I appreciate work is not always an environment that you can control and sometimes you work through your lunch break but it is worth trying to make time during your lunch break to eat as mindfully as possible. Managing to do it three times a week will still be a big step forward from what you may be doing now.

If you have a lunch room or anywhere outside, take yourself away from the work environment and sit there. You can talk to colleagues, even if it is about work, as long as you make sure for those 15 minutes or so that are spent eating, eating is the main focus of your mind. The danger is that you forget you've eaten lunch and then reach for something else soon after. If you do this, it is likely to be a type of food you need to eat quickly, perhaps something from a vending machine, which increases the chances it will be unhealthy and high calorie.

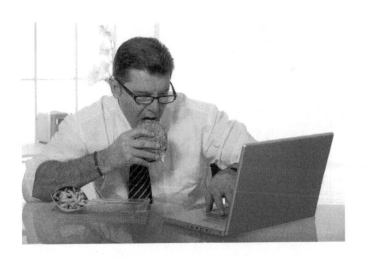

© Depositphotos.com/marcomayer

If you can try and get into a routine and let people know that you want to take time out to eat your lunch, it will make it easier. I am sure it's more difficult in some jobs than others but whatever you can do to allow yourself the necessary time to properly eat your food will help you get the most from it.

Conclusion

- Try and identify your established habits that need to be changed in order to support your goal of a healthy weight. Think of the changes that you would make. Be open minded, don't forget what your goal is here; you need to prioritise. Some will be easy, fish and chip Friday can still take place but instead of the chip shop food you can steam some cod and peas and have some oven chips.

- Start setting the table and eating at it. Make it an enjoyable experience that allows you to focus on the food and not unconsciously move the food from your plate to your mouth. The only thing that you should be staring longingly at during a meal is either your food or your partner, not any sort of screen!

- Get into a routine and stick to it. If you know you definitely can't eat at the table one day, make sure you do another. Try three evening meals at the table in your first week.

Chapter 7

Thursday Big Shop

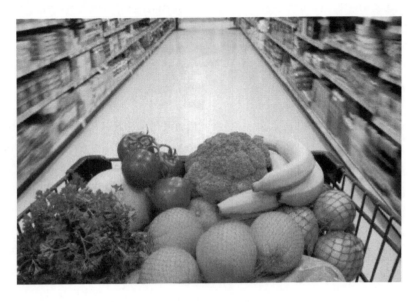

© Depositphotos.com/mikedon

The Thursday big shop in our house was something I always looked forward to. My mum hated shopping at the supermarket and my brother and I were hardly keen on it, so it fell to my dad to do the weekly shop on a Thursday night. By the time Thursday came around everything had run out and only the crackers in the kitchen we left for snacks. I particularly liked the fact that my dad used to get a strawberry cheesecake for me and the minute he got home I would rifle through all the bags looking for my glorious treat. I'd then eat it in a particularly mindless way before he'd even started to put the shopping away.

Whether you do a single shop each week or whether you go several times a week, 100% of British people visit the supermarket at least once a month[1]. The supermarket is king when it comes to giving us the food produce that we want to buy. The problem is, though, that while some of our main concerns are budget, health and weight management, the chief concern of the supermarkets is to make you spend as much money as possible by buying as much produce as possible. Reconciling the opposing goals of us and the supermarket is no easy task, which could go some way to explaining our nation's health crisis. So, how do we make sure that when we shop at a supermarket, we buy what we want and only what we want?

One option is to not shop at the supermarket and shop at local shops and other individual outlets such as markets and farm shops. For many people, this isn't practical; one reason for the dominance of supermarkets is the convenience factor of having everything in one place.

We buy a lot of what we buy because of our habits. How often do you go to the supermarket and start at the same produce, then follow the same route around the supermarket, going up a particular aisle or down another one and have a pretty similar basket or trolley to last week? It's especially easy to buy the same things when you shop online as you can repeat order things and if you forget, the website will remind you that you ordered a 12 pack of beer last week but for some reason have not ordered this week. They, of course, can add it automatically for you.

The average supermarket stocks around 25,000 products, but the average household uses only 300 different products a year and only 150 on a regular basis. This is a good example of established habits in our shopping. Perhaps part of the reason for this because people don't have time to learn how to cook different foods or perhaps they're really happy with their diet and don't want to change anything. If you ask yourself whether you are happy with your diet, what would your answer be? If you're not happy with your current diet, then you need accept that your 150 products that you regularly buy from the supermarket are going to change.

It's common knowledge that we shouldn't shop when we're hungry because we end up buying more. There are plenty of other reasons why we buy more than we planned to at the supermarket. Here are some statistics from various studies and research experiments:

- Quick trips to the supermarket can result in buying up to 54% more food than you planned[2]

- Impulse buys can account for between 50% and 67% of all purchases depending on your social demographic[2]

- Baskets mean less impulse buys than trollies[2]

- You are presented with a special offer every one and a half seconds

It's clear that the supermarkets win the battle in getting us to spend and buy more than we'd like to.

Shopping Strategy

How exactly are we to regain control of our purchasing and only buy the things that we want?

The first step is to know what it is that you want because if you do know what you want, the supermarket will decide for you. The best way to work out what food and drink you want to buy is to sit down and work out what you're going to eat. It will take no more than an hour to work out what you're going to have for the week, you have 21 meals to plan, plus snacks. Most people will eat a similar breakfast each day and usually have a similar lunch. Lunch can also be an extra portion of the evening meal so you don't have to plan 21 individual meals, you probably only need to plan 11 or 12 at most, and that's allowing for 2 different breakfasts, 4 different lunches and 6 different evening meals. If you have children it might up things slightly but even if it takes you an hour and a half, it's a very well spent 90 minutes. You will also want to write down snacks and other incidental items that you might be wanting to include in your diet over the next week. Doing your thinking now means you can think less later, when perhaps time is tighter.

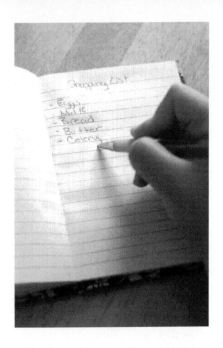

When you spend this hour working out what you're going to eat you are introducing a system that provides some control over your diet. Make sure you're not starving, not too stressed and not rushed so that you can rationally work out what you really need. One reason for this process is that you're making the decision about what to eat while you're state of mind is neutral. If you shop for food while you feeling a particular emotion in a strong way, e.g. anger, it's likely you'll over eat, eat unhealthy foods and eat more often than if you are shopping with a plan and a strategy. I know several people who call at the supermarket on their way home from work and their emotions influence their buying choices. They are stressed so they throw in some chocolate or a double pack of doughnuts because they deserve it after a hard day's work. They are rushed and late so they just grab the quickest available option for their evening meal, perhaps a ready meal or a pizza or something.

By spending time planning your weekly shop when your mind is neutral, you are taking some of the risk factors out of the shopping.

The point of this exercise is to build a list, the list which forms the backbone of your supermarket shop. If you go without a list, you are banking on your memory, someone phoning you whilst you're there or plain old luck as to whether you're going to get a balanced shop. You're also giving carte blanche to the supermarket marketing team as they love nothing more than an indecisive shopper with an empty trolley to fill.

You might think this a methodical approach to buying food from a supermarket, but don't forget you want change, and this is one of those changes that will help you achieve your goal. Once you change the way you do things, previous habits that weren't conducive to a healthy weight are removed and new habits, which do help you successfully manage your weight, are formed. When you have developed habits that support health, you don't need to think about it as much, because they become established habits. So there's a short term investment (habit change) for long term gain (established healthy habits). The reason why we want an accurate and complete list is so we control the purchases and not the supermarket. I'm going to discuss some of their methods to influence your purchases in the next section.

Super Marketing

I said earlier that we're presented with a special offer every 1.5 seconds. I'm not approaching this section with the aim of saving you money, although you may just do that, I'm approaching it with the aim of helping you to control your purchases and not buying foods that won't help with weight management or over buying foods.

Not So Special Offers

I want to talk about the different types of offers that supermarkets present you with every time you walk through their doors.

x for £x

This is a very common offer and it works because it suggests a number for you to buy, for example it could be 2 for £3 or 3 for £5, so if you weren't sure just how many you wanted, now you are! Sometimes the saving is insignificant but the supermarket plays on the fact that the special offer signage will get your attention, the very fact it is an offer will push you into buying and the suggested quantity you purchase will guide you in how much to buy.

Limit of x per person

This type of offer implies that there is some scarcity in the product being sold and that if you don't get yours now, they'll all be gone. In fact, it's such a good offer that we're having to limit you to 12 per person! These offers are particularly enticing when it is something that isn't perishable and will keep for a long time. The sales difference between "Sale, 99p" and "Sale, 99p, limit of 12 per person" can be huge, all because they've limited the quantity you can have.

Multipack

The signage for multipacks and multibuy are generally the same colour, font and shape as the special offer signs, where there is actually a price reduction. We have come to associate bulk buying and multibuys with saving money, but in many cases it isn't true. You might get 4 in a pack or 10 in a pack or perhaps it's a larger container, but often they offer no advantage over the smaller equivalents.

Having some knowledge about how supermarkets work is useful from a financial perspective, but my main aim is not to help you save money. There are lots of other good books out there to help you do that. My main aim is to prevent you from over buying so you don't over eat. Supermarket offers such as the ones I've listed can increase the amount you buy by between 30% to 105%[3]. Most people buy one or two of their chosen items but offers either suggest to you or explicitly tell you how many to buy. In the case of x for £x and multibuy, they are telling you exactly how many to buy, even if the saving's are very negligible or even if there's no saving at all. In the case of the limit of x per person offers, they are suggesting a number to you so you up your limit from one or two and put in five or six.

If you're sceptical about whether these kinds of offers can influence you or not, you can look at some of the studies carried out. Everyone likes to think that they make their own decisions but there is a reason why the supermarkets have these offers, nothing is accidental or random, and the reason they have them is because they work.

Have a look at the offers below, they are some of the offers I've talked about it and they seem very catchy. Like many offers, though, the saving is hardly worth it and ironically in these offers, you don't make any saving at all.

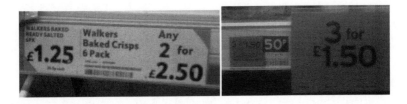

Next time you look at an offer, try and work out if it's really worth it, from a financial perspective and a weight management perspective, don't trust the supermarkets to get everything right.

First Line of Defence

The reason I don't want you to over buy foods is

because once they come into the house, you're much more likely to eat them. Say you usually have a box of cereal in your cupboard and they were on special so you bought three. You now have three boxes of cereal in your cupboard. What this has done is brought you away from the norm, which is one box. It's very hard to not do this, but what automatically happens is that you want to return to the norm and so you start to eat more of the cereal so you can get back to the norm of only one box. How many times have you run low on milk and so you use a little bit less to try and make it last? The reverse is true, if you have loads of food in the cupboard, you'll have more and eat it faster because you think there's a huge surplus. This is especially true if you ram it all in the cupboard so everything is a mess and the only way to sort the cupboard out and get it tidy is to eat some of the food.

One way to help deal with this is to store the extra food in a separate place such as a pantry or garage, to try and prevent you from thinking you can have huge portions without making a dent in your stocks.

So the first line of defence is represented by your shopping, if you don't buy it, it's not in the house and if it's not in the house, you can't just eat it as you're passing through the kitchen or feel a bit bored and start rummaging through the cupboards.

Name's Not Down Not Coming In

The single most effective way to ensure that you do not

buy food that you don't need is to use a list. We've already talked about the importance of planning your food ahead and the result of that is a list. If you make a list and stick to it, you won't buy unnecessary food. Everything you need is on the list, because you've planned your meals so if crackers are 3 for £3, you can ignore it because you don't need them as they're not on your list.

Nine out of ten of us make impulse buys and on average we visit the supermarket three to four times a week, so there's a lot of opportunity for impulse buys. Making a list gives you purpose, you don't need to wander around the supermarket trying to think about what to eat on what night because you've already done you're thinking in your planning session. This means you won't be wondering about what to buy, waiting for the supermarket to make the decisions for you and steer you in the right direction.

I appreciate that some offers are very tempting and sometimes you can save a fair bit of money by buying in bulk. Generally, though, most offers aren't helpful for your weight management because most offers are geared towards bulk buying. I'm trying to help you manage your weight, which is not helped by buying large quantities of food.

Overbuying any food isn't a good thing but as many offers are geared towards unhealthy foods, it can be a double whammy.

Before something goes into your trolley, you must ask yourself why it's going in. Your list contains the food that is going to make up the meals and snacks over the next 3 days, 7 days or however many days you've made the list to cover. If you buy a packet of biscuits that isn't on the list then they're going to sit in the cupboard or biscuit barrel. And they will call to you. Until you eat them. Add up the calories in the extra biscuits and you've given yourself a lot more work to do to lose any weight.

It's important to have a policy that says anything not on the list does not enter your trolley or basket. You need to stick by your list because this what is going to be the barrier between you and the seductive offers of the supermarket.

Carrying Bags

One strategy for making sure you pick up only what you need is to limit how much you can carry. Think about the last heavy snow we had and how you shopped for food. I walked to our local supermarket with a rucksack and had to be selective as to what went in it. I wasn't in a position to carry back 12 cans of lager, 8 pints of milk and a load of potatoes. Instead, I selected what I needed and nothing else because I knew I had to carry it back home. Had I selected unnecessary and unhealthy foods, I would not only have had to carry them home in my rucksack, I'd have had to carry them on my body after I'd eaten them!

Walking to the supermarket with a rucksack or a bag on wheels means you get some exercise but you also need to think about what you're buying. A list can help because a few chocolate bars might not weigh much but we don't want them sneaking into your bags.

If you drive to the supermarket, take a basket rather than a trolley, because then you can use that as a reference for how much to buy and be equally selective as to what really needs to go in there. Take a trolley and you can just load it with unnecessary and impulse purchases because you'll have no trouble fitting it into the car to get it all home!

Conclusion

- Do not underestimate the influence supermarket offers can have over your buying habits. The supermarkets would not adopt the strategies that they do if they didn't work, even if we think we're the ones who can't be influenced.

- Your time spent planning your strategy and your meals can make a real difference to how much you buy at the supermarket. The time spent making your list is time well spent because you're taking control of your purchases.

- If making a list and being aware of how influential supermarkets can be allows you to reduce over buying by even 50%, it will be a very worthwhile process.

Chapter 8

Reading Between the Labels

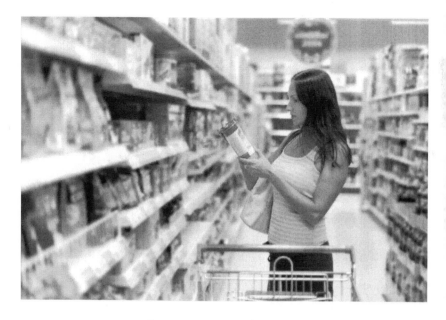

© Depositphotos.com/xxxpatrik

I want to talk about the labels that we see on foods, because it's useful for you to understand them and interpret them in a way that's going to help you successfully lose and manage your weight.

Before I get in to anything, I want to give you an idea of the approximate amounts of energy, sugar, fat etc. that you should be eating every day. Individual needs will vary based on build, weight, activity levels and other external factors. The figures below are the current government recommendations.

	Women	Men
Energy (calories)	2,000	2,500
Protein (g)	45	55
Carbohydrates (g)	230	300
Sugar (g)	90	120
Fat (g)	70	95
Saturated Fat (g)	20	30
Fibre (g)	24	24
Salt (g)	6	6

This will now give you a basis for understanding the rest of the chapter. The reason I want to dedicate some time to talking about food labels is because it can be complicated and because it can make a big difference to your diet.

There are two main reasons for food packaging looking the way that it does on a particular product.

1 - Make the product appealing for sale

2 - To comply with legal obligations

Notice there is no "3 - Provide useful and easy to understand information to the customer"! Make no mistake, packaging is designed to make you buy the product and to ensure that the manufacturer and retailer are legally meeting their minimum requirements.

As packaging is not designed in your best interests, I want to give you back some control so that you can make your own decisions with the correct information and not be influenced by packaging.

Energy Density

While it's certainly true that we overeat, it's not just the quantity of food that is worth pointing the finger at. The quality and specific content of food is also another important area that can help weight management.

Food gives us energy and if we take 100g of any given food, there will be a certain amount of energy in that 100g of food. The British Nutrition Foundation classifications of energy density are as follows:

Very low = < 60 calories per 100g

Low = 60 - 150 calories per 100g

Medium = 150 - 399 calories per 100g

High = > 400 calories per 100g

While I agree these classifications are helpful, I think that the medium category should be altered, so they classifications read:

Very low = < 60 calories per 100g

Low = 60 - 150 calories per 100g

Medium = 150 - 249 calories per 100g

High = 250 - 399 calories per 100g

Very High = > 400 calories per 100g

The majority of what we eat should be low energy dense foods, with very low being the next most eaten group followed by medium, with high and very high being an occasional food and eaten in small quantities.

The reason I propose a new category is because foods with an energy density of 350 calories per 100g would be classed as a medium energy dense food so it gives the impression that it is something that can be eaten quite liberally. These foods are not something I would encourage so readily, particularly when attempting to lose weight or manage your weight.

The energy density of the average British diet is 160 and the recommended energy density for a healthy diet is 125 calories per 100g.

So if your diet consists mostly of foods such as bread, crisps, snack bars, fast food, restaurant food or convenience foods, it's likely that the energy density of your intake is more than your energy requirements.

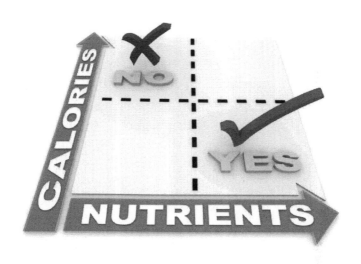

Confusion

I bet you can name at least five foods which are supposedly healthy but would fall into the high or very high energy density category. Does this mean you shouldn't eat them? Not necessarily, and here's where it gets complicated.

Whole grains are a recommended source of fibre and because they release their energy slowly, are an important component of a health diet. Whole grains, though, fall into the high category for energy density, so, what does this mean for someone trying to lose or manage their weight?

Oats, pasta, wheat, brown rice, beans, quinoa, and barley are all foods that have a high energy density. When you eat these foods, you are generally going to eat them with something else, unless you're a pasta freak, you will probably have something other foods to make up your meal. If you are eating your pasta with vegetables and some chicken or beef, the energy density of the overall meal will reduce as the vegetables will balance out the pasta. This would mean that the energy density for that meal falls into the low to medium range, which is great.

If you had porridge oats for breakfast, you could swap some of the oats for an apple, lowering the energy density of the meal.

Other foods such as nuts and seeds will feature in the very high energy density range. These are an important part of your diet but you only need a small amount every day. The reason that these are important is because many essential vitamins and minerals are contained within each little nut or seed. These are what we call nutrient dense foods. So we only need a small amount of them and because we are only eating a small amount, it doesn't matter about the energy density being really high.

Foods such as pastries, cakes, biscuits and crackers fall into the very high category for energy density. Their nutrient content is low, so these foods aren't actually required at all and eating them regularly can make a big difference to the energy density of your diet.

The rough guideline is to make the average energy density of your entire diet falls into the low category. This will be an average because you'll want some of the nutrient dense very high energy dense foods and you'll balance that with plenty of foods that are low to medium in energy density.

To illustrate the point, two studies have been done showing how much the average person eats in a year. One had a figure of 1,500lbs, the other 1,996lbs. I'll user the lesser figure to be conservative.[1,2]

If I eat 1,500lbs of food per year and it has an energy density of 200 calories per 100g, this means I'm eating 3,731 calories a day. If my energy density was 140 calories per 100g, my calorie intake would be 2,612 calories per day. If my energy density was 120 calories per 100g, my calorie intake would be 2,238 calories per day.

So you can see that the energy density of your food can make a huge difference to your calorie intake. The difference between an average energy density of 120 calories per 100g and 140 calories per 100g is over 135,000 per year!

So being aware of energy density and aiming for most of your foods coming from low / medium energy density foods will help you maintain a healthy weight.

Traffic Lights

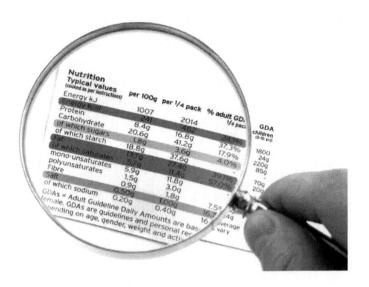

© Depositphotos.com/brianajackson

The government has introduced a standardised traffic light labelling system in 2013. The actual presentation of the labels may differ between different retailers, but the information and colour schemes should allow the comparison of different foods. The sugar, fat, saturated fat and salt content are all highlighted in a different colour. Red means high, amber medium and green low.

SERVES 2 - HALF PIZZA PROVIDES				
CALS	SUGAR	FAT	SAT FAT	SALT
495	9.0g	18.3g	9.2g	2.00g
25%	10%	26%	46%	33%
OF YOUR GUIDELINE DAILY AMOUNT				

The picture above gives a label from a pizza and the pizza serves two people so we are given the traffic lights per serving. What if I want to compare it against another pizza? If the pizzas are different sizes, it's impossible to compare servings as one pizza might contain more fat but it might actually be a much larger pizza, how do I know if it's better overall or not?

The comparisons should be per 100g rather than per serving, as different foods have different serving sizes, so always compare based on 100g of each food (or 100ml or drinks). Many foods now have traffic light information per 100g as well, to make comparing foods easier. Often, though, this is on the back of the packet and requires you to look for it rather than having it easily presented on the front (remember what I said about the packaging not being there for your convenience?).

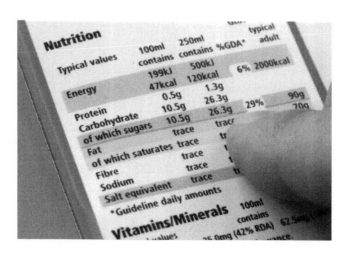

© Depositphotos.com/brianajackson

The picture above shows a the label from a drinks carton and you can now see the nutritional information per 100ml, which means you can compare like for like with other drinks and then make your decision. This example does not use a universal traffic light system but has the retailer's proprietary system, which is also colour based using different colours and more categories...helpful.

Red, amber and green may be easy to understand at a glance, which is good, but it's not always as simple as that.

Confusion

There are limitations to this system, which are useful to be aware of in terms of food choices and weight management.

If you just ate everything that was green and ignored everything that was red, you'd be excluding whole food groups from your diet, which wouldn't be a good idea.

In order to be eating a balanced and healthy diet, a bit more detail is required. For instance, high fat foods such as nuts, milk and fish may be rated red for fat and cause people to avoid these foods. The fats in nuts and fish are healthy and are essential to the body. Avoiding these foods could lead to a deficiency in omega 3 fats.

Fruits could be classified as high sugar under the new labelling scheme, even though fruits are a perfectly healthy and essential part of any diet.

The most important item on the labelling system is sugar, as sugar represents the biggest cause of weight gain in many people. The common advertising message that retailers have used in recent years is "Low fat means weight loss" and they backed up their advertising with low fat products that could be bought as an alternative to the original product.

The problem is that people see "Low fat" on a product and buy it based on that alone, why would you buy the high fat product if you can have low fat? One main reason added fat is in our foods is because it increases flavour so if you remove it, you either lose the flavour or swap the fat with a flavour replacement. So the manufacturer has swapped fat for chemicals or sugar to increase the flavour whilst keeping fat down.

The low fat message has not worked because fat isn't the main offender, sugar is the guilty party and if you only look at one part of the label, look at the sugar content.

Muller Light Yoghurt is a good example, the "Light" is prominent on the label and the fact they contain fruit is also easily readable for the customer. The issue for me is the ingredients and the nutritional information and how this relates to the packaging.

Firstly, you'll notice how prominent the "Light" is. Incidentally, the word "Light" means there's a similar product with higher fat. Oil with 95% fat could still be classed as light if there's an oil with 97% fat on sale.

Secondly, look how much fruit is displayed on there and

how much yoghurt. Much more fruit than yoghurt I think you'd agree. Yet this is misrepresenting what's actually inside, as the yoghurts are only 10% fruit.

Thirdly, there's a picture of a heart on the packaging and inside it says it's fat free, which implies it's good for your heart. It might be fat free but they still put other things in here that they aren't so proud to shout about.

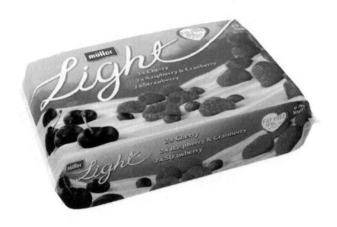

The ingredients and nutritional information are: "Yogurt, Water ,Strawberries (10%) ,Fructose ,Modified Maize Starch ,Gelatine ,Flavourings ,Beetroot Juice Concentrate ,Acidity Regulators: Sodium Citrates, Citric Acid ,Stabiliser: Pectins ,Sweetener: Aspartame"

Typical Values	Typical values per 100g
Energy	217kJ 51kcal
Protein	3.9g
Carbohydrate	8.1g
of which sugars	7.1g
Fat	0.1g
of which saturates	0.1g
Fibre	0.2g
Sodium	0.1g
Calcium	120mg

So we have an almost fat free product, which sounds too good to be true! Which, of course, it is. It might have no fat but your yoghurt will contain 14.1g of sugar as well as an artificial sweetener (which, incidentally, is 200 times more sweet than sugar), and this begs the question of how sweet do they want it?!

The fruit content in this particular yoghurt is 10%, but clearly that's not enough fruit to colour or flavour the yoghurt adequately as the manufacturers have also added flavourings to flavour it to taste like strawberries and beetroot juice to make it appear as a strawberry colour.

So making low fat foods an integral part of your diet is not really a strategy that's going to give you positive results. Any food is an acceptable part of a healthy and balanced diet, even foods that are red on the labelling system, but these should not constitute the main part.

The below guidelines apply to food content and the information that can be stated on labels:

	Low (g per 100g)	High (g per 100g)
Total Fat	<= 3	>= 20
Saturated Fat	<= 1.5	>= 5
Sugar	<= 5	>= 15
Salt	<= 0.3	>= 1.5

Notice that the threshold for low fat is less than three percent. Notice that the value for high far is 20 percent. So while you may see "Low in fat!" plastered all over the products, it's rare that you see "High in sugar!" displayed quite so prominently.

There's an awful lot more that I could talk about with regards to food labelling, manufacturer claims and ingredients that most people would rather not be in their food, but this book is about weight loss and weight management rather than an informational about the food industry. The main thing I wanted you to take from this was that in future you could benefit from being more aware about labels and taking a bit more time to read between the labels to see beyond the marketing.

Conclusion

- Be aware of the content of foods, particularly paying attention to the amount of sugar you're consuming

- Don't take the manufacturer's claims at face value. "Low fat" and "Lite" usually means that sugar and other stuff has been inserted into the food in place of the fat

- Just because a food has a red traffic light does not mean it should be avoided. Common sense can still be your best guide, fruits and nuts are still essential, cakes and chocolate need to make up only a small part of your diet

Chapter 9

Successful Portion Control

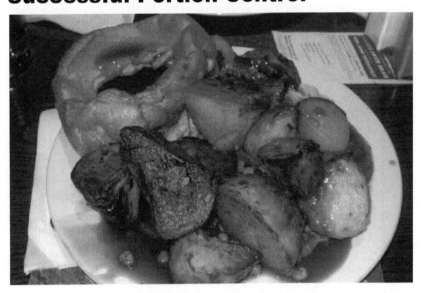

Have you ever been to a Toby Carvery and watched in awe as people plate up their foods and carry the resulting mountain of food back to their tables? Christmas dinner is another good example of overloading a plate, particularly if my mum is plating up. Five different kinds of vegetables, three different kinds of potatoes, stuffing, Yorkshire pudding, apple sauce and, of course, a pound each of turkey. It's all lovely but how on earth am I supposed to eat all that?

Christmas dinner might be a once a year event but think how much food you eat at meal times. The process that is used to get food from the fridge or cupboard to the plate can either work to support weight loss or weight management or support weight gain. I'm going to talk about that process from beginning to end to help you identify any changes that might be beneficial to you.

My mum used to cook Sunday dinner every week and it was basically Christmas dinner without quite so much variety and without the best crockery. When plating up, my mum would ask me how many potatoes I wanted, how much veg I wanted and how much apple sauce and stuffing I wanted. She'd then serve that amount and sneak another 20% or so on top of that, presumably because she wanted to make sure I was fed. Even if I couldn't finish all of the food, I still ate more than I would have done because it was on my plate and that meant my rating on the hunger scale, which should be a 7 ends up being a 9. I'd over eaten.

How you plate up your food and how you arrange your table can affect how much you eat. Assessing your hunger and taking a mindful moment can help prevent unnecessary eating but if you are hungry and having some food, it's still possible to overeat. I want to talk about some of the things that can lead to over eating in a single sitting and what can be done to avoid them.

Portion Distortion

Portion size is something that is relevant every time we eat or drink. Our needs as humans have not changed that much in the past few thousand years, but the amount of food we eat has changed and so have our portion sizes. I just want to list the suggested serving sizes of some commonly eaten foods:

- Kellogg's Bran Flakes 750g - 30g with 12ml milk

- Pringles 190g tub - 30g

- Tesco Margherita Pizza 335g - one half of pizza

- Tesco spaghetti 2kg - 75g

As an example, when you're having your breakfast, which may be your chosen cereal, how much do you think you serve? Do you think it's near the 30g that the manufacturer suggests? Do you think you have around about 125 of milk? And do you only have 75g of spaghetti or do you just pile it into the pan? And when you have a pizza, do you have the whole pizza or just half like the suggestion says? It's surprising how badly we estimate how much is a suitable portion. I'm going to talk about the factors that can influence how much you serve yourself and then talk about how you can use these influences to work in your favour.

Container Size

The size of the container you are serving from influences how much you can serve. One study was carried out in with people divided into two groups. One group went into a room where they were presented with snack mix served in two containers, each capable of holding a gallon. The other group went into a room where they were presented snack mix served in four half gallon containers. This was the same amount of snack mix, just different containers. The group taking snack mix from the larger containers served themselves 53% more than the group taking snack mix from the smaller container and they ate 59% more than the other group.

Another study was done in which people served themselves ice cream. Some people served into 17 ounce bowls, others into 34 ounce bowls. The people serving into the larger bowls served 31% more. Even the size of the ice cream scoop made a difference, with the bigger scoop resulting in more ice cream being served.

So the size of the source container, the size of the serving utensil and the size of the target container can influence how much we'll serve ourselves. When we serve ourselves, we will eat at least 90% of what we serve.

To tip the balance back in our favour, we need to make sure that we're serving from a reasonably sized container and it's going onto a reasonable sized plate or bowl. This isn't easy, though, as plate sizes have risen from an average of 10 inches in 2002 to 12 inches in 2012. This two inch addition gives the plate an area that is 44% larger, and who ever leaves loads of room on a plate? On average this leads to an increase in calorie intake of 22%. [1]

Measure the diameter of your plate and unless it's 10 inches or smaller, I would advise getting new ones so you avoid over filling your plate.

If you've bought a huge container full of food, such as cereal or pasta or something, you can split into multiple plastic containers so that you're not serving yourself from some monstrous container.

Get a big saucepan out and you'll boil more potatoes to make it look full. But you can also use this to your benefit by using it in reverse. If you are cooking vegetables, use a big pan so you will have a tendency to cook more.

If you're not sure what 50g or what 100g looks like, weigh it out. Use the same storage box, bowl or plate as you would do normally and then once you have a rough idea what these quantities look like, you should be able to do it by eye from then on. Weighing food for every meal is going to be overkill and not really practical but doing it once or twice so you can get your reference point is a worthwhile exercise.

Eating Out

If I offered you a drink in a pub, take away or a restaurant what would you have? Would it be a small, medium or large? What about if I offered you a portion of chips, would you have small, medium or large? You might be shocked when you get what you've asked for and find that one or two sizes down would have been enough - who can manage a venti at Starbucks?!

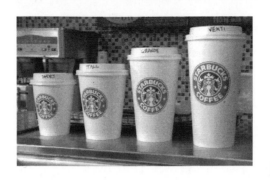

Your idea of small, medium or large may differ entirely from the sizes at the restaurant or take away place where you are. Many people might say small if they're not hungry or thirsty, medium if they're neutral and large if they're quite hungry or thirsty. Rather than answer straight away, ask them to show you and tell you how much is in each type of container. Many retailers have now discontinued small, renamed the previous medium to small, renamed the previous large to medium and introduced a new version of large. They keep the name small but they've upped the size every single container, upping the size means upping the calories.

Usually, eateries size their containers on the big side, so you might get a surprise if you order without seeing the amount you're going to get. Try ordering one size down from what you normally order and see if you can tell a difference. Once you've ordered it, you're more likely to eat or drink it because you've paid for it and it'll be sat there right in front of you.

Value

One crucial influence over how much we eat is the value of food, or at least, our perception of the value of food. For example, the table below shows some details of McDonald's chicken nuggets. It's common for many places to price food so that the more you buy, the cheaper it becomes per portion.

	Calories	Price	Price per nugget
6 Nuggets	250	£2.69	45p
9 Nuggets	375	£2.89	32p
20 Nuggets	835	£4.49	22p

Here, you can see that if you buy 20 chicken nuggets, you get each nugget for half as much as if you buy 6. If you perceive the value to be better if you buy more, there's a chance you'll over buy and therefore over eat. It's the same as when you buy a coffee from Costa or a sandwich from Subway, the larger serving you buy, the cheaper per millilitre or per gram it becomes. Some chains run "Meal deals" where the cost of a sandwich and drink separately is the same as the "Meal deal" cost, which is a sandwich, a drink and a packet of crisps. The crisps are free, so you may as well have them as not having them would be like throwing money away. Pizza Hut offered an upgrade from a medium to a family pizza, for free! So I get more pizza for the same money, which sounds good, but is that really good for me? Great if you're having a pizza with a family but if you're on your own, they're offering you more calories and more fat in the same meal, maybe on second thoughts, it's not such a great offer for you.

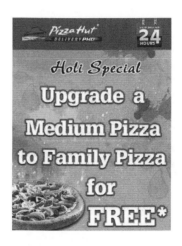

Getting the best value for your wallet is a good thing and in today's climate, is something that all of us should be doing. If you're looking to lose weight and change things, though, you should be looking to get the best deal for your body. The best deal for your body does not always match the best deal for your wallet, particularly when eating out. Eating well does not have to be expensive but there is a reason why the absolute cheapest food is commonly the food that is the least healthy.

If the shop tells you that you could have a packet of crisps for free, you can say no or give them away. You don't have to eat them just because they are part of some special promotion. If 9 chicken nuggets works out cheaper than 6, you don't need to eat 9. You might be getting better value but you're still spending more and taking in 50% more calories.

Upgrading to a Subway footlong from a 6 inch sandwich can be only 47% more expensive yet you are getting 100% more product[2]. This works out at better value for your wallet but less good value for your body. You're getting double the size of your sandwich so is a 53% saving in cost worth a 100% increase in calories?

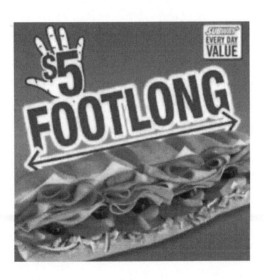

Variety

Have you ever had a box of chocolates and had to have about 6 in one go so that you can sample all the flavours in the box (except the coffee one, obviously)? Do you think people would do the same if there was only one flavour in the box? Do you think someone would eat the same amount of food at an all-you-can-eat Shepherd's Pie night or at an all-you-can-eat buffet night? There are lots of examples where variety of either foods or flavours can increase our intake. Imagine an ice cream shop that sold just vanilla ice cream, how many scoops would you have? One, perhaps two? What if they had 36 flavours, then what? I'd bet most people would have at least three.

When people in a study were offered three flavours of yoghurt compared to only one, they ate 23% more.

Whether it's colour, shape, flavour, type or the number of containers you are serving out of even if the food inside them is the same, studies have shown people serve themselves more.

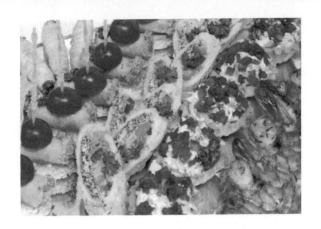

When you're cooking, try not to give yourself too many different options in the same meal. This particularly works when you're at a buffet, a carvery or a party where there are nibbles. There is so much variety and you want a little of everything. Be aware of how much you're putting on your plate so you don't fall into the trap of over loading because you want to try it all.

Make it work for you by having multiples types of vegetable but only one type of potato or starchy carbohydrates.

Total Food

The total amount of food you prepare can be related to serving size. For example, who says a serving of minced beef is 400g or 500g? If you have made your list you should know how much food you want for each meal. If you over cook you are likely to over serve and therefore over eat.

Leaving leftovers on the table is a sure fire way to increase the calorie intake of your meal. Leftovers should be left in the kitchen, that's why they're called leftovers. They are not required so you leave them. It is not a reserve in case you couldn't fit enough on your plate the first time. A meal on a 10 inch plate should be plenty for most people. If you over cook, leftovers may not be enough for another meal so you may face a decision between throwing in the bin or eating. Neither of which are ideal situations.

Cooking in meal multiples will help reduce any leftovers and reduce the chance of over eating. As you have made your list, you'll know how much food you need per meal and then you can cook in multiples of that, so cook one or two meals at once, rather that one and a half, which encourages over eating. You'll minimise the risk of ending up with not enough food for another meal but too much food for one meal. This involves planning but leftovers can really add unnecessary calories to your diet.

Appearance

Appearances can be deceptive, which is why you need to deceive yourself into thinking you are eating more than you are. When I was working in an office, I would take two sandwiches to work, both wrapped in tinfoil. One I'd have around 11:30 and one around 13:00. The sandwiches were from the supermarket "Freshly baked" bread section and I'd have four slices, two for each sandwich. It was a loaf so you had to slice it yourself (I couldn't deal with those slicer machines) and when I sliced it myself, I'd make a mess because the slices would rip or be uneven. The only way I could get consistent slices was to make the slices HUGE, they were three quarters of an inch thick. The seven or so guys in the office all marvelled every time I ate one of these sandwiches. It probably worked out that 90% of the sandwiches were bread, and it probably worked out around 700 calories in the bread every day.

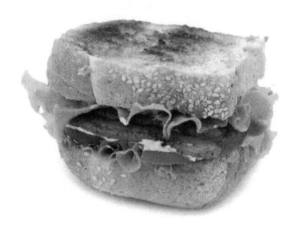

© Depositphotos.com/geniuslady

Realising this wasn't a great strategy, I stopped doing this and decided to replace the bread with salad and other fillings such as tuna, egg or cottage cheese. I added a lot of salad leaves and increased the amount of other salad ingredients. If I wanted a slice of bread, I would still have that but even with the giant slices, it was still cutting the bread calorie intake by a three quarters. The important thing here, though, is that I did not feel deprived or had some expectation that I wouldn't be full because the volume of the food was still the same. I just bulked it up with nutrient dense food rather than calorie dense food. Plus, it was a lot easier to eat as trying to get a sandwich the size of dictionary in your mouth isn't easy and doesn't do much for the professional image when everyone at work is sat watching the rather graceless spectacle!

If you are making any foods, whether it be a one pot meal, a sandwich or spaghetti bolognese, try increasing foods that take up physical space but are low in calories and losing a bit of the calorie dense foods such as bread, spaghetti, rice etc.

If you're buying lunch and you see a sandwich with what appears to be lots of filling, prepare for disappointment as you realise that 80% of the filling has been disproportionately moved towards the visible side of the sandwich to make it look fuller. After a couple of bites you are usually just eating bread. The big baguettes you can buy from the sandwich shops are mostly bread, so while you think you're getting a sandwich, it's basically a baguette with little goodness and lots of calories.

Making the sandwich yourself or buying a salad that contains some meat or beans that will fill you up is a better idea than a sandwich where 85% of the calories come from bread.

Serving Method

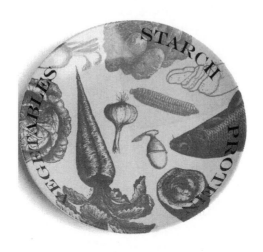

How you serve your food can influence how much you're going to eat. A good strategy for putting the food on your plate is to have half of the plate covered in vegetables and the other half equally split between starchy carbohydrates or protein. The vegetables must be put on to the plate first so that you don't overfill with carbohydrates and protein and have no room left for the vegetables. From a weight management point of view, vegetables are a great help because they will fill you up and they have low calories, sugar and fat. They are also nutrient dense and energy sparse in terms of what you get in return for relatively few calories.

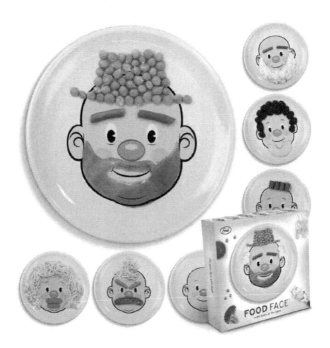

You can even buy plates that have the proportions printed on them to remind you of how to portion up your plate. These can be really useful in encouraging and learning good habits. These plates can be useful to encourage consistent portioning but if you fancy a bit more fun (though admittedly, much less useful) try the Food Face plate. Make every mealtime a fun time! Two halves of a green bean probably doesn't constitute a portion of vegetables, so stick with the portion control plates! But if my wife is reading this, I think I know what I want you to get me for Christmas!

When you serve, serve from the kitchen and then take your food laden plate to the dining table to eat. If you have a kitchen diner, leave the saucepans on the side. You want to sit as far away as possible from whatever you cooked the food in. If the saucepans or trays are left in sight and within reach, it's so easy to keep topping up your plate as you go along. You don't need seconds, if you had cooked exactly one portion each, you wouldn't have finished eating and then rushed back to the hob to start cooking more, would you?

Lost in Digestion

I mentioned in the chapter on Hunger that we can eat up to 28% more when the reminders of what we've eaten are cleared away[3]. Not every food leave a reminder on the table but there are some foods which do, and these reminders are useful, so they should be left. It could be bottles of beer, chocolate wrapper, chicken bones, crisp packets, drinks cans or the toothpicks from the mini kebabs you get. If there's anything available to remind you of how much you've had, leave it on the table so you don't forget and overeat.

Eating With Attitude

One of the attitudes that is extremely common is that we must always clear our plates. Two thirds of American parents still urge their children to clear their plate, whether for a reason given above or for some other reason, but this is not a helpful approach when it comes to adult life. These attitudes and beliefs stay with us for life and can be hard habits to break. It's likely that we'll then pass them on to our own children and the problem then perpetuates. These attitudes and beliefs are drilled into us as kids thousands of times (three meals a day for 16 years) and we forget the internal cues of our body and rely on the external cues like the empty packet, clean plate or time of day.

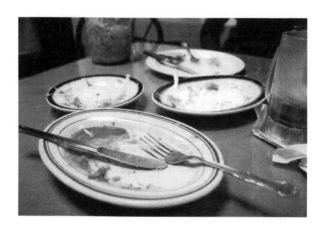

The first thing to mention about that is I might not always want exactly the amount on my plate. I might not always be one plateful hungry or I may find the food very filling and I am satisfied with only three quarters of what I've been served. The clear plate belief is a bit of a double whammy if too much has been served in the first place as you're not only clearing your plate but you're clearing an overloaded plate. Why is clear your plate so popular?

• Children starving in third world countries - "There are loads of children in the world who would love the food you've left on your plate"

- Someone has paid for that food so don't let it go to waste - "Me and your mother go out and work hard to buy the food we put on your plate"

- You are a growing child - "You need to build your strength, get it down you"

- You don't want to offend someone by leaving food when they ask you "What was wrong with it?"

There may be children starving in areas of the world who would indeed enjoy the meal on your plate. The truth is, though, whether you eat the last two roast potatoes won't make a difference to that situation. You can do other things to make a difference but whether you clear your plate or not doesn't change things, even if you might feel slightly better because of what you were told as a child.

It may well be that you paid for the whole tin of beans and hate to see the last bit go to waste but how is eating something you do not need any better than throwing it away? If you throw it away it goes in the bin and will biodegrade with time. If you eat it, it will be stored as fat on your body for you to carry around with you. That sounds quite wasteful to me. Both throwing in the bin and eating unnecessary food are wasteful but if I had a Yorkshire pudding left on my plate that I didn't need, I know I'd rather end up in the bin than stored on my body as fat.

You are indeed a person who needs to keep up your strength and energy, but this can be done by eating in accordance with your body's requirements, not overeating.

You can leave some of the food that they've cooked for you if they've cooked too much. You can tell them how nice it was and how satisfying and how you would like that meal again in the future. You don't have to make your body feel uncomfortable and stuffed to bursting just to make someone else feel better.

A message of clean your plate is encouraging you to push yourself until 9 or 10 on the hunger/satiety scale. How many times have you pushed yourself to cram in the extra few chips on the plate, even though you were already full? You then sit back with a sigh and let out an "Ahh" as if you've achieved something special.

The clear your plate rule does not stack up and it's not an effective way of eating. Changing your plate size and planning how much to cook can all help in preventing an overloaded plate from making its way onto your table. At least then if you clear your plate, you're only clearing a reasonably sized and reasonably loaded plate rather than an oversized and massively overloaded plate. It's important that you eat mindfully and are in touch with what the needs of your body are, this should override all other cues.

I do not like waste, I'm sure most people would agree. The way to avoid waste is to not cook it in the first place and the way to avoid cooking unnecessary food is to not buy it in the first place, which means planning your meals. Have a look at the flowchart below, which shows the basic process of how food gets from shop to plate.

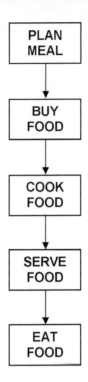

PLAN MEAL

↓

BUY FOOD

↓

COOK FOOD

↓

SERVE FOOD

↓

EAT FOOD

You have to make decisions that affect potential waste earlier in the process. You don't have to do down to the nth degree in terms of planning how many potatoes each person wants but you can do rough calculations, i.e. 4 people at 3 potatoes each means 12 potatoes as opposed to half a bag or whatever method you may have used previously. If you do end up cooking too much you could save some for another meal rather than topping up the plates with what's left in the pan. This way you haven't served the extra so you know that food won't be wasted, either thrown away because no one could finish it or it being unnecessarily eaten.

It won't prevent all waste, though, but it will minimise it. If you can't finish your plate because your hunger is satisfied, that's OK, in fact that's perfect because you have demonstrated that you are in tune with your body. It is important to understand that you don't need to finish every thing on your plate or everyone else's plate to feel at ease. Unnecessary food entering your stomach or the bin is waste, so don't think by eating it, you're helping yourself or avoiding waste.

Conclusion

- It's very easy to allow external factors to control how much you eat, whether eating at home or eating out and about. You need to switch on your brain and be consciously aware of what's going into the pans to cook or what you're going to order.

- Prioritise things to support your weight goals. The better value in terms of money may not be better value in terms of health, make sure you buy what you want and what you need, not what the restaurant or sandwich shop want to sell you.

- Switch your bowls and plates to a size smaller so that you don't over serve yourself. Check the sizes of food when ordering out and order a size down. If you eat and drink mindfully, you won't notice the size difference.

- Plan your meals so you don't massively over cook or over serve. This will help you minimise waste. The primary aim for every meal should be to eat until your body is satisfied, not to eat everything in sight.

Chapter 10

Will You Not Have A Nice Cup of Tea?

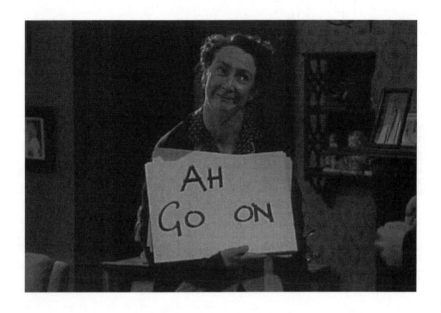

If you watched Father Ted, you might remember a character called Mrs. Doyle. She was the housekeeper who was intent on making sure that the priests were well fed with cakes and well replenished with tea. Her method of making sure the priests and guests sampled her food and drink was to ask in a gentle way "Will you not just have a nice cup of tea?", to which the guest would reply "Ah, no thanks Mrs. Doyle, I'm not really thirsty", to which Mrs. Doyle would then reply with "Ah go on, go on, go on, go on, go on, go on, GO ON!" and then the guest would finally relent and have a cup of tea, to Mrs. Doyle's delight.

Why did the guest have the tea, we know he wasn't thirsty, so why did he say yes?

Have you ever done something similar?

Can you think of any time that you've eaten or drank something someone else has offered when you didn't want it?

- Your Mum when dishing up Sunday dinner?
- The in laws?
- The host of the B&B you're staying at?
- The person who's birthday it is at work?
- Someone who offered to buy a round at the pub? The host of the party you are attending?
- Why did you say yes when you meant no?

It's common in people with weight issues to be very bad at saying how they feel, particularly when it comes to saying no to food offered. This is generally combined with low confidence and assertiveness levels. There are so many situations where unwanted and unnecessary food can be offered and this makes it an important consideration in weight management. I want to say early on that I'm not saying you should refuse every bit of food or drink offered but you need to know how to do it otherwise you'll be swamped with offerings from well meaning people. One particular characteristic of offering other people food and drink is that it is generally associated with cakes, biscuits, crackers, alcohol and other unhealthy items. I call these people Food Forcers, because they like to quite literally in some cases, force their food into our mouths.

Here are a few common reasons that we accept food we don't really want:

- We don't want to offend the other person

- We want to get on the other person's good side

- We want to have one because everyone else is having one

- We don't want to be different

- We don't have the confidence to say no

- We don't know how to say no

- We say no, they insist and we say yes

- It's an established habit, i.e. Giant Yorkshire puddings for Sunday dinner at Mum and Dad's

There are a few possible reasons why the other person might be so insistent that we take up their offer:

- They want to be seen to be friendly and hospitable

- They want to show dominance by changing your mind

- They might not really be listening to any objections

- They don't want to be rejected

- They think you are just shy and really do want it, even though you're saying no

- They want you to take up the offer because they've spent time making the food/drink

- They want your feedback on their cooking

- They might want you to fail at your weight loss because they've failed at theirs

All the reasons above for someone insisting that you accept their offer are all to do with THEM. This person wants your feedback, they want your gratitude, they want to feel like they are a good host, they want to feel kind and they want to feel like you need them. It's all for them, not for you. I know it sounds harsh to say this about someone offering you some food but often they're not doing it for you, they're doing it for them. It is very true that it's better to give than to receive. The fact they are offering you something is laudable but it is important to remember the bigger picture of a) whether you want it and b) whether you need it.

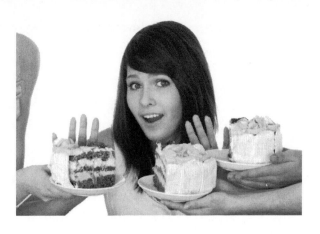

We need to get the focus onto you. Can I interest you in a cigarette? Go on, it'll make you feel good? Just one tiny puff, you'll like it, I promise. OK, if you really don't want it, just have it for me, then. You don't know you'll like it until you try, just give it a go. Go on, go on, go on....you get the idea. Are you getting tired of saying no yet?! People can be persistent, can't they? With this example, I bet you would have been able to refuse because I imagine you would have said "No thanks, I don't smoke" and that would be the end of that. You turned it from something about them into something about you. Considering most people can quite easily refuse someone when offering us cigarettes, alcohol or drugs, why do we find it so hard to refuse food?

One explanation is that food has, for most of our lives, been an expression of love and kindliness so refusing it is snubbing someone and risk hurting their feelings. In order to effectively refuse food, you need to make it about you. If the other person is offended, that is their problem and it is their decision to feel like that. The responsibility to keep them sweet is not yours, it is theirs.

The best way to deal with offerings of plenty that you don't really want is really simple and it involves you saying "No thanks, I don't want any". That's it. No explanation, no regret and no additional information. You do not have to justify your reasons. If the person does a Mrs. Doyle and repeats the offer or even more forcefully and tells you to accept, just repeat yourself with a polite "No thanks, I don't want one" or "No thanks, I'm fine without". It's really important you get the result you want rather than letting someone else control your food or drink intake.

If you're thinking this is too hard and you won't be able to do it, don't worry. This is a natural initial response, no one likes refusing hospitality and when they do, people generally like to give a reason so the host doesn't feel bad. You could say "No thanks, I don't want any, but it looks delicious" so you have given them a compliment to soothe their disappointment.

Try and practice this aloud to get used to saying it. Be in front of the mirror so you can see how you look and gain confidence with telling someone that you don't want something. Find a friend and do some role play to practice refusing what you don't want. This is a skill and comes with practice, so don't be concerned if at first it seems difficult or awkward. Don't forget, someone is offering you food or drink to be kind but also for their satisfaction. If it's an apple or a small glass of wine, it's probably not a big deal but if they're offering you a slice of their lovingly homemade high calorie cake or a glass of the tenderly put together yet high sugar punch, it's not necessarily OK. Your weight loss and weight management goals trump all and nothing should be allowed to get in the way of it. If they are offering you something that is going to make your main goal, you're super important life changing goal, more difficult than it already is, you should have all the reason and motivation you have to politely refuse. With NO explanation!

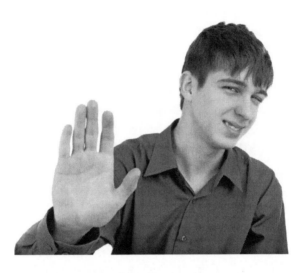

© Depositphotos.com/sabphoto

"I'll try it later" is lying, "Just a small bit" is copping out and "Oh, go on then, one won't hurt" is letting someone else make the decision for you and giving them the impression you'll cave in so they'll put on more pressure next time. The responsibility for everything that passes your lips is your own, don't give it away. I just watched

Top Gear with Jeremy Clarkson and he was challenging James May to a race in New Zealand. Clarkson in a car and May in a boat. Clarkson said he had chosen the fastest car in the world for this challenge, which turned out to be a humble Toyota. It wasn't just any Toyota, it was a rented Toyota. He said he could push it to the limit, crash it, drive as fast as he wanted to and the reason for this reckless attitude was because the car does not belong to him. Clarkson was OK as he had collision damage waiver insurance, you don't have the equivalent for your body.

Have you ever been round to someone's house and because that person is hosting, they've prepared a load of food. They don't want to look like bad hosts, after all.

One thing I like to do is ask if they are going to have some, to see what they say. I have often had the reply that they are not hungry or they say what my Mum says at Christmas; "These are for guests so I won't"

Does that mean I could host a party and say that I'm not eating much but I'll offer you 3 pints of lager, 2 glasses of punch, a huge portion of quiche, lots of crisps and nibbles and some ice cream and cake to finish?

Why do I offer you all these food that I can't eat myself?

Because your body isn't mine. I don't care if you have one or fifty, I just want you to eat what I've made and look like you're enjoying yourself. Your weight goals aren't going to affect my life but they will most certainly affect yours.

By letting someone else make the decision about what and how much you eat, you've given away responsibility. This is when you enter the casino of weight loss because it's totally random as to whether you'll succeed or not. Don't forget, when you enter a casino, it's not usually you who wins! Add to that the possible guilt and anger you'll feel afterwards and it's better for everyone if you politely refuse what food or drink you don't really want.

If you often find a friend or family member who is playing the role of food forcer, explain to them beforetime that you are losing weight, you are taking more care of yourself and you won't be eating things that you don't want to eat. They should understand, but if they don't, it's going to be more fun saying no to them! You should not have to give ANY reason for your decisions but if you really think you're going to struggle with the "No thanks, I don't want any, but it looks delicious" approach, then giving people a heads up is a good way of preventing the problem occurring.

Eating Out

When you eat out, you're opening up to the possibility of taking on many more calories than you think you are and taking on loads more than you really need. Part of this is due to the established habits that we talked about earlier and part of this is because eating out means someone else is going to prepare your food so you don't have the control or the knowledge of what's going into it. Choosing a restaurant that is more likely to have dishes that are healthier is a good part of the strategy. Italians may have some good pasta dishes and most do white meat and fish dishes as well.

British food will have healthy options such as white meat, a vegetable hotpot or a lean steak but there may also be pies and battered fish on the menu. Indian and Chinese dishes tend to have a high fat and calorie content, so you'll have to be wary of what you're eating if you go to these places. The national chains generally have their nutritional information online, so it's useful to check it out to give yourself a good insight into the nutritional value of your meals.

When ordering from the menu, you can order exactly what is written on the menu or you could ask them to change it to the way you would like it. You obviously don't have control over every aspect of the food but there are things you can ask the chef to alter, things which don't take much effort but can make the dish a bit more healthy, a difference sometimes worth making.

The chef does not care about health, they care about making the food look appealing and making it taste nice. What makes food appealing and taste nice? Oil, sugar and fat. This is what they're going to put in the food to make sure your taste buds like it. Plenty of oil, sugar and fat isn't compatible with weight loss, which means you need to either choose a dish low in these or you can ask the chef to lessen the content. Since you are paying for the food, it's not unreasonable to ask for the food how you want it. I commonly give the waiting staff loads of instructions about how I want my food so I get what I want. It seems a shame to pay money to eat out only to have food that would have been nicer if you'd have prepared it at home. Here are some of the things I ask:

- Can I have the dressing/sauce on the side?

- I don't want any oil

- Can you go easy on the cheese?

- Is the beef used in the meatballs lean?

- Is the soup cream of tomato or just tomato?

- Can I swap the roast potatoes for boiled?

- Are the chips oven baked or fried?

- Can I swap the onion rings for extra vegetables?

- Do you do a fruit salad for dessert?

- Do you have wholemeal pasta?

- Is the tuna just tuna or is it mixed with mayonnaise?

- Does the chicken have the skin on?

- Is the sauce a cream or cheese sauce or is it tomato based?

- Are the vegetables steamed or are they pan fried with butter?

- Is the pizza on a thin crust or is the crust quite thick? (Health concerns when ordering a pizza, I know...)

In fact in one restaurant I went in, I couldn't find a main course I wanted and I ended up having three starter dishes instead. They were happy to oblige since I was a paying customer.

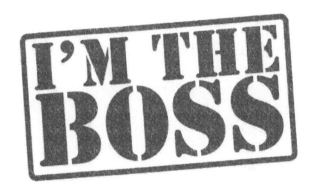

© Depositphotos.com/chrisdorney

There are lots more questions you could ask to find out more about the food you're paying for. If you find out what you're getting before hand it's much better, you can make changes then. If you wait until the food is in front of you, there's more chance you'll eat it, so pre-empt any issues by talking to the waiting staff beforehand.

Other strategies for ensuring a meal out doesn't result in excess intake are:

- Have plenty of water before the food arrives

- Miss out a snack earlier in the day, but don't skip a meal

- Have a salad as a starter (watch the dressing, though, as it'll be high in fat)

- Try and avoid the all you can eat buffets

- Start eating last and pace yourself to be level with the slowest eater of the group

- Be aware of the calorie and sugar intake of the drinks you are ordering, these can sometimes add up to more than the food

- Ask yourself if you really need dessert, coffee or the mint at the end of the night

- Ask yourself if you really need the large portion, even if it is only 20% more in cost

- Check what the meal comes with before ordering side orders. Once it's on the table, there's more chance you'll eat it

- Let other people have the bread and push it to the other side of the table or ask the waiting staff to remove it

- Cut the fat off the steak or try and have leaner sources of protein

- Remember that pasta, rice and spaghetti carry plenty of calories

- Ask for a cordial and soda to drink and ask them to make it weak to reduce the sugar

- Try and keep the company of people who don't have weight issues or generally eat less than you do

- If you weren't going to ask for it if there is no reason why you should eat it just because they did offer

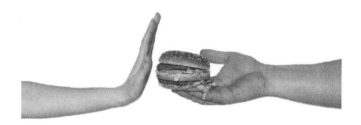

Conclusion

- Try to understand how important it is to make sure that you get your own way when it comes to the food and drink that you take in.

- There's no reason why a party, a get together, a meal out or a barbecue or any event must mean that you consume a lot more calories than you wanted to. One dessert, one pint, one deep fried haddock won't make you put weight on but all of these things on a regular basis will have an effect on your weight, particularly if you're in the weight loss phase.

- Don't make it harder for yourself, don't risk feeling guilty afterwards, don't look for someone else to blame afterwards, instead, just use the polite refusal and polite requests to make sure that you get what you want and I promise you will be glad you did.

Chapter 11

Weight Loss Makers & Breakers

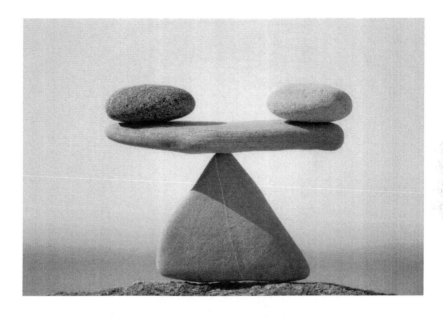

© Depositphotos.com/styf

There are other aspects to your diet that can make a big difference to your weight loss and weight management efforts. We're going to look at those areas now.

Snack Attacks

The definition of a snack is "A small amount of food eaten between meals". Snacks are a common part of most diets and most people have at least one or two snacks a day so the difference they can make to calorie intake is considerable.

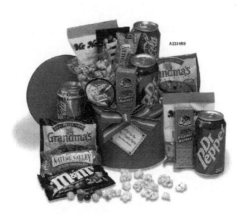

A snack for many people could generally be something like one or two pieces of fruit, a packet of crisps, three crispbreads or biscuits, a cereal bar, a handful or two of nuts or small tub of yoghurt etc. There was a time for me when snacks used to consist of HobNob biscuits, a Mr. Kipling apple pie, a home made bun or a packet of Skips crisps. My problem was that I would not just have one of these things, I would have loads. The problem with having big snacks is that they result in you taking in loads of calories and the amount of calories can often exceed those of a meal.

Snack maths: too many snacks = a meal

A piece of fruit, a chocolate bar, a packet of crisps or a biscuit or two are all reasonably sized snacks. These are all snack type foods and you might be eating them at a common snack time such as 11am or 3pm. I've known several people who decide to eat two chocolate bars or two packets of crisps and because they are eating the snack foods and snack times, they still consider that particular nibble as a snack.

Too many snacks will give you the same calories that you find in a meal, even if the physical size of the snack is less. The definition of a snack then becomes "A meal sized amount of food eaten between meals" - clearly this is not a good strategy and research shows that snacks can contribute to weight gain. To demonstrate this, consider the below:

Four McVities HobNob biscuits weighing a total of 56g give you 268 calories.

One Mr. Kipling apple pie weighs 66g provide 229 calories.

A Marks & Spencer tuna and three bean salad weighing 355 grams gives you 355 calories, although without the dressing it is similar to one apple pie or the HobNobs.

So you get over 5 times as much food for pretty much the same amount of calories. Snacks may be little in weight and size but they make up for it in calories, fat and sugar.

There are some ways to minimise the damage that will be done by snacking.

Don't snack - do you really need the snack? Have you assessed your hunger and had a Mindful Moment? It may be possible to avoid the snack altogether, perhaps go for a short walk and reassess in 10 minutes.

Eat less of the same snack - having a glass of water before snacking can help increase satiety and therefore you could eat less of the snack but still feel the same as if you'd had your usual portion. Try having a glass of water and then waiting 10 minutes to see how that affects your snack intake.

Eat the same amount but swap the snack - a snack swap means replacing the sugary high fat snacks with something like crispbreads, oatcakes, nuts, yoghurt, fresh fruit or a low sugar cereal bar. There are lots of good alternatives out there that don't provide a huge calorie intake in one go.

Drinks

Drinks are often overlooked as contributors to daily calorie intake. Many people consume a wide variety of drinks from squashes, bottled juices, energy drinks, hot drinks, alcohol and soft drinks. Squashes, bottled juices such as J20, energy drinks, hot drinks such as hot chocolate and coffee, soft drinks and alcohol can contain significant quantities of calories, fat and sugar.

The examples to the below are averages, not the maximum content in their class. For example, a Starbucks Mocha Cookie Crumble Frappuccino (with whip) Venti with whole milk contains 566 calories, 19.8g of fat and a barely legal 89g of sugar!

	Cals	Fat (g)	Sugar (g)
Carlsberg draught lager 1 pint	182	0	0
Starbucks Standard Caffe Latte Tall, semi skimmed milk	143	5.1	12.8
Red Bull 250ml	113	0	27
Fanta Orange 330ml	160	0	44
Aero Instant Chocolate 24g	97	1.8	13.9
J2O Apple & Mango 275ml	74.2	0	17.05

These figures really do surprise people because they don't associate drinks with bad health. There's a common trend where people drink energy drinks because they believe it will give them more energy. What really happens is a huge sugar rush followed by a sugar low, and what do you need when you have a sugar low? An energy drink. It's a yo-yo cycle that can devastate your weight loss efforts.

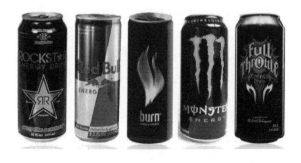

Sports drinks are also a popular choice for people, but unless you're actively participating in sports, they contain calories and sugar which you won't use for energy. Drinking Lucozade Sport might make you feel like an athlete but if you're not actually doing these exercise part of the deal and you have a 500ml bottle, you've just added 17.5g of sugar to your daily total.

Alcohol is another calorie powerhouse, containing 7 calories per gram. If you have just one pint of lager a night, you've added 1,274 calories to your weekly total. Spirits represent a better option than lager or beer but reduction of intake is the best option.

Reducing the size of the drink you order will help you reduce your calorie intake. You can also pace yourself and make sure you don't drink too fast to avoid ordering more drinks to make up the difference. Ordering beer or lager in half pints, ordering short sizes in coffee shops and removing the optional extras such as whipped cream and sprinkles can make a difference.

You could try halving the amount of drink you have and topping up the rest with water. You still retain most of the taste but you've halved the calories and sugar. You can apply this technique to all sorts of drinks from squashes, fresh orange, energy drinks, sports drinks and the pre made fruit drinks.

Diet alternatives are available, although some of the sugar substitutes they use are less than perfect, from a weight loss point of view, these are a better, if not ideal, choice.

Water

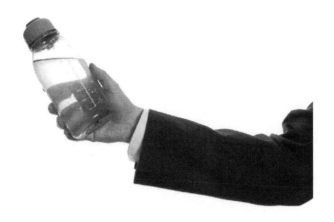

© Depositphotos.com/yanc

Often overlooked as an aid to weight loss and weight management, water is the most important nutrient for the body. Your body is two thirds water and water is required for many essential functions that you need from day to day. Water contains no calories so it's a great choice for a drink, especially since lack of water can turn a healthy body into an unhealthy body.

Water contains potassium, calcium, magnesium, fluoride and sodium, so is itself a source of many vital minerals. Water is essential in transporting many other nutrients around the body.

Water is involved in eliminating toxins from the body in the urine and water is the primary constituent of sweat, which is another mechanism for eliminating toxins from the body. Without this mechanism, the amount of toxins in the body can become too high.

If the body is dehydrated due to lack of water, symptoms can occur, such as fatigue, headaches, hypotension, irritability, constipation, dry mouth and eyes, light headedness and if the condition becomes more severe joint problems, cholesterol problems and a weak pulse can result.

The symptoms of dehydration can often be mistaken for other things and you may find yourself reaching for an energy drink of a chocolate bar to try and give yourself an energy boost whereas what you really needed was hydration from water alone.

From a weight management perspective, we've already talked about how water can help with satiety and preventing over eating. Having a glass of water can help remove any feeling of hunger altogether and watering down popular drinks can help reduce the sugar and calorie intake.

To get more intake of water, buy a good 1 litre bottle that has measurements on the side and have it at work on your desk, this will help you to keep track of how much water you are drinking.

Drinking 2 litres a day should be your aim, although tea and coffee doesn't count towards your intake, in fact these can cause you to need more water.

Condiments

Condiments, sauces, dressings and dips can add calories and fat to your diet. They seem insignificant because they aren't really the main part of your meal but they can really add up.

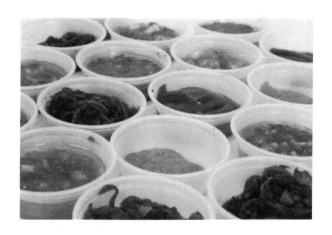

© Depositphotos.com/yupiramos

Coleman's Classic Mint Sauce is 23% sugar, while their Apple Sauce is 25% sugar, Hellman's Light Mayonnaise has 27g of fat per 100ml, Mary Berry's Light Salad Dressing is 27% sugar and 22% fat, Parmesan cheese is 28% fat and Old El Paso's Sour Cream dressing is 28% fat. These are high numbers for someone actively trying to lose weight and it's important to be aware of them if you're trying to manage your weight. When you're adding these kinds of things to your meals, it's important you understand what kind of impact these can have on your overall calorie, fat and sugar intake.

You may want to avoid them completely as your food doesn't really need them but certainly I would recommend as small a portion as you need to minimise the increase in calories.

Planning

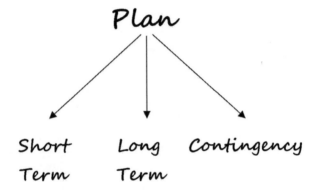

There are a lot of suggestions in this book about how you can change things in order to successfully manage your weight. Some these things, such as your time spent planning meals and shopping lists take time, which many of us are short of.

When you plan, it's because you want to know the answer to a question or know what to do before you have do it. This saves you making a decision with no time to think or having other factors influence your decision. If you're going for a job interview, you don't just turn up and see what happens, if you really want the job you spend time predicting questions and working out your best answers. You could just turn up and see what happens to your weight, (I'll give you a clue; nothing) or you can predict things, plan things and work out the strategy for your course of action.

Short Term Planning

Short term planning involves thinking about the current day or the next day. This means thinking about what you're going to have for lunch, what exercise opportunities there are, thinking about tea etc. etc.

This could involve making your lunch so you can take it to work with you rather than having to rely on the staff canteen or sandwich van. Marks & Spencer have some healthy salad lunches but they will become expensive if you have these on a regular basis. The cheapest form of healthy food is that which you make at home. So short term planning involves you making your lunches, packing your snacks into conveniently sized bags or containers, making sure you have a water bottle to hand and getting a meal out of the freezer after you get home from work. If you know you are going to be spending the day without somewhere to get a healthy lunch, it's important to take one with you to prevent an impulse decision brought on by hunger and convenience. The result of these is often a visit to the vending machine or canteen, which don't often have healthy choices.

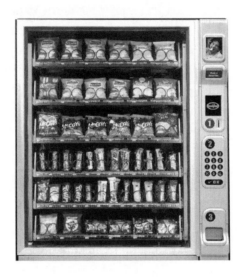

A packed lunch and your prepared snacks means you are controlling your dietary intake for that day. This is a much better approach than having to make do with what's available during your day.

Making sure you have enough food in to make your snacks for the next day is essential, so if you are running low, you can call at the shops on your way home from work. You can also pick up anything that you need for your evening meal, to avoid reaching for the frozen pizza or dialling for a takeaway.

It is also important to consider when you might make time for your physical activity. Planning this in advance means you are more likely to do it rather than getting to the end of the day and having no time.

Some of these things mean you might have to get up half an hour earlier or go to bed half an hour earlier. Perhaps you can do two things concurrently and use your time more effectively to allow yourself time to make your meals of go for a walk. If this is what it takes to maintain a healthy diet and regular physical activity, then I would hope you think it is worth it.

Long Term Planning

Long term planning is thinking about the coming week. Your meal planning session before your supermarket shop is a good example of long term planning. Making sure you have the food in for your evening meals, the food in to prepare your lunches and snacks for work, sorting out your physical activity times and reshuffling depending on work or social commitments are all examples of long term planning. You want your week to run smoothly and the best way to make sure that happens is to plan.

If you're going out on Friday night, you might want to get your physical activity in on Friday morning or early evening so you don't have to do it on Saturday. You could make sure you have a good and healthy evening meal so that you aren't tempted to snack when you're out.

If you're going to be busy all Wednesday night, make two packed lunches and double the snacks so that your busy Wednesday night doesn't affect Thursday's food.

Contingency

There are always times when you haven't had time to plan your food properly or make the necessary arrangements to ensure you have the food you want for that day. This should not be a regular thing but circumstances can occur that mean you are left with options that you don't really want.

In order to avoid these situations occurring, you need to have a contingency plan for when you run out of options.

Your snack drawer at work can still be a snack drawer, just with a few alterations from a traditional snack drawer. In there you can keep some low sugar snack bars, some tinned fruit, tinned soup, packet of oat cakes, a packet of Ryvitas, packet of nuts, a couple of John West Light Lunches and some plastic cutlery. This means you've got some snacks and some meals for when you have no prepared food and haven't got time to go out or aren't able to get a healthy option. Your contingency means you can still maintain your healthy eating that day. You can keep the same set of food in your car, a small box in the boot, so that you always have something, even on the road. You probably won't have an in car microwave for the soup but the John West Light Lunches should suffice. Add a couple of bottles of water, though, and you'll be self sufficient without having to rely on service station food.

Remember, this is all to stop you having to make rushed and poor decisions because of a lack of preparation and a lack of options. It will also stop you eating food you didn't really want and feeling bad that you may have ruined your diet for the day. I've already talked about dealing with setbacks but preventing the setback in the first place is a better option and that's what you'll be doing here.

Conclusion

- Employ the Mindful Moment before your snacks to tune into your body. Be aware of how much you're having to control the snack portion

- Use your new knowledge of what drinks really contain to reduce your intake. Watering down is a really good way of doing this. Alcohol can make weight loss and weight management a real struggle. Ordering a size down, alternating between water and alcohol or swapping for spirits can help reduce the calorie intake.

- Plan effectively by making sure that your needs are taken care of and that you have a contingency in place for those times then you weren't able to prepare food yourself.

Chapter 12

Exercise to Support Weight Loss

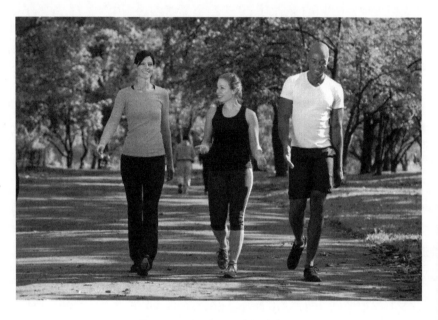

© Depositphotos.com/simplefoto

Your overall health and weight loss efforts are going to be between 70%-80% diet related. The remaining 20%-30% will be down to your activity and exercise level. There are clear links between sedentary lifestyles and many conditions ranging from obesity, depression and even premature death.

In the UK, only 40% of men and 28% of women meet the recommended levels of exercise for adults. The government recommendations for exercise are:

• Everyone should do a minimum of 150 minutes a week

of moderate-intensity aerobic exercise but that really is the minimum for health benefits. If you can go beyond 150 minutes, you'll gain even more health benefits.

- The intensity at which we exercise is key, and light activity such as strolling and housework is unlikely to have much positive impact on the health of most people. For aerobic exercise to be beneficial it must raise your heartbeat and make you sweat.

- Sedentary time (time spent sitting down to watch TV, use a computer, read or listen to music) does not help your health, even for those who are achieving 150 minutes of exercise a week.

The fact that so many studies show so many links between inactive lifestyles and conditions that you don't want to have, shows that exercise is an important part of any lifestyle. This doesn't necessarily mean going to the gym every day but being active, i.e. moving about, I'll talk more about this later. We know exercise is good for us, but let's take a closer look at some of the benefits of exercise:

1. Helps weight loss by burning calories

2. Lowers blood pressure and improves your cholesterol and triglyceride levels

3. Improves your insulin sensitivity and reduces risk of diabetes

4. Heightens your mood by releasing endorphins;

exercise is a proven antidepressant

5. Reduces the risk of cardiovascular disease, heart attack, stroke, high blood pressure, cancer and many other diseases

6. Strengthens your heart so that it doesn't have to work so hard

7. Increase your stamina and endurance, meaning you will be able to do more and feel less exertion

8. Enhances your immune system, reducing the risk of common colds and other illnesses

9. Helps the mind focus and helps your attention span

10. Regular exercise will add years to your life

Calories and Exercise

Exercise burns calories, which is good news.

This means that you can help your weight loss efforts by exercising to burn off the excess weight that you have. In order to best support your weight loss efforts, it is useful to know that you must create an energy deficit by using more energy than you create. You can't destroy energy, this is the law of the Conservation of Energy. You cannot create or destroy energy, you can only change it from one form to another. In our case, we are talking about changing the energy provided in food to energy you will then use in activity, or, in the case of taking on too much energy, the form will be changed so that it is stored as fat, ready for use. The energy that you have stored can't be destroyed, it needs to be changed from one form to another and exercising will turn that fat into energy, which you will then use. To lose weight, you need to create an energy deficit, so that you are using more energy than you are taking in. For your weight management approach, you keep the energy in and energy out round about level.

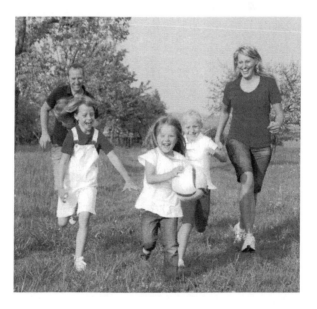

© Depositphotos.com/kzenon

One fact that surprises many people, though, is just how many calories you need to burn off to negate the effect of a chocolate bar or a packet of crisps. The amount of calories that are used when exercising depends on the type of exercise, the duration of exercise and the intensity of the exercise. Modify any one of those and you can really alter the energy used. Your weight and genetics will also affect how many calories you use when exercising.

If we take a person weighing 15½ stone/100kgs/220lbs who eats two scoops of ice cream, they will have to walk at 3mph for 31 minutes or swim for 11 minutes to burn the same amount of calories as they consumed in the ice cream. If they ate a 30g chocolate bar, that's 27 minutes of walking or 10 minutes of swimming. Two slices of pizza, depending on topping and crust could mean you have to walk as much as two hours just to burn off those calories! This illustrates just how important activity is in terms of helping to increase your energy expenditure, and when you add in the added health benefits, exercise and activity is something that should be incorporated into your lifestyle.

Exercise Ideas

Physical activity does not have to mean spending hours in the gym every day or exercising to the point of exhaustion.

There are lots of ideas to get the 150 minutes per week recommended for health benefits. It is likely that when you find something you enjoy, you will do more than the 150 minutes per week.

Go for a walk - sounds obvious but so many people do not do this. Walking is so easy and accessible to many people and really can make a difference in terms of weight loss and raising the heart rate to provide health benefits.

Do some gardening - even if you don't have a garden, you could offer to mow the gardens of any elderly neighbours. You will do a good deed and get some exercise.

Wash your car - this is a good way to get active and you can volunteer to do any neighbour's cars. Again, you do a good deed as well as getting yourself active.

Walk to the supermarket - walk to the supermarket with a couple of bags or a rucksack. Even if you have to make two trips, this is a great way to get some exercise into your routine.

Walk the dog more - if you haven't got a dog, volunteer to walk someone else's. You can do them a favour as well as giving you a good reason to get out and walk. The dog will thank you as well!

Walking round the park - you can get your walkman (I'm old fashioned) out and give yourself a target of walking for three, four, five songs or even an entire album. This will help you progressively build up your time.

Make an activity day at the weekend - hire bikes, follow a hiking trail, go to a swimming pool, go to the park and play a game with the kids - anything to get you moving.

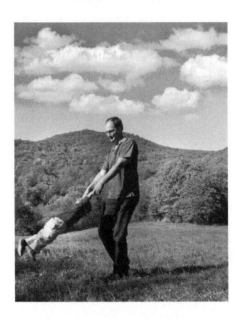

Arrange to do whatever it is with somebody else, perhaps join a group or a class. This will make it much easier to incorporate into your routine.

Daily Activity

The NHS talk about something called Active Daily Living (ADL). This means integrating activity into your everyday life. Notice the active in activity, this means you need to move! Watching TV, driving, sitting and watching football or going to the cinema don't count as activity, they are not active tasks!

I want you to make a couple of lists. One list will be made up of your incidental activity that contributes to your Active Daily Life. This could be cutting the grass, walking the dog, vacuuming, washing the car etc.

I then want you to make another list of deliberate activity that makes you a bit sweaty or out of breath. This could be swimming, walking or hiking, or an exercise class of some kind.

What do your lists look like? Is one longer than the other? Are they both the same size? Are they long or short? When you add up the amount of time you regularly do these activities, does it work out at 30 minutes a day or more? 30 minutes really is the minimum to support any weight loss or weight management programme.

You don't have to do the entire 30 minutes in one go, you can break it into 10 minute segments throughout the day. This is achievable for almost everyone and even if you haven't found one of the suggestions that is agreeable to you, there will be things for you.

Meeting the minimum requirements for exercise will give you benefits but exceeding them will exponentially increase the benefits for you. Aiming for 45-60 minutes 5-6 times a week with at least two of those sessions which would be targeted exercise making you a bit sweaty and uncomfortable. You'll get benefits in terms of health, fitness and weight loss so it is worth acknowledging and embracing the fact that exercise is an important part of any weight loss or weight management programme.

Conclusion

- If you want to give your weight loss efforts the best possible chance of success, making the time for activity and exercise is an important step, one that can't be missed out. If you go above and beyond the minimum recommendations then you will receive benefits beyond weight loss as your body responds to what you are asking of it.

- A healthy lifestyle includes being active and doing some exercise. If you think that this is too much effort then you are not after a healthy lifestyle. You may be after your version of it, but it will be a version without those amazing benefits that exercise brings. If you ask nothing of your body, your body won't give you much back. Your body can do a lot more than just sit down all day so start asking more of it!

- You should know by now that I don't care about excuses. Whatever excuse you have, there'll be someone with more reasons not to exercise and more barriers to overcome who does ten times the exercise on your list, so know that nothing can stop you!

Chapter 13

Successful Implementation

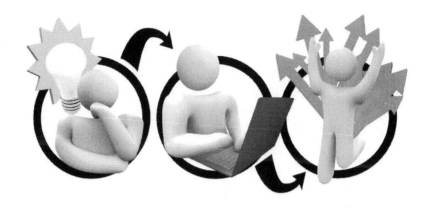

© Depositphotos.com/iqoncept

This is it, the last chapter! You might be feeling satisfied with yourself by making it this far but you've only just begun. Reading a book is the easy part, now you've got to go and put it all together.

I have provided you with a lot of information that will help you alter the way you eat, the way you drink and the way you interact with food. There are lots of techniques and advice I have given you, which when implemented, will make a big difference to your diet, reducing overeating, making you more aware and giving you control of your actions.

Some things might require you to be slightly outside your comfort zone, they might be a new concept to you and you might not be sure about how it will work for you. It's important that you still try things, with your fullest effort to ensure that you give yourself the best chance of success.

If you just cherry pick the easy bits and miss out the stuff that takes effort, you are not going to succeed and not succeeding because you only gave a half hearted effort is not acceptable. What do we tell our kids when they get 16 out of 20 on the spelling test or didn't quite make the football team? Even though we wanted them to get full marks and make the team, we tell them we are proud of them as long as they did their best.

Doing the easy bits does not constitute a proper attempt. And the results will reflect this.

Why would you want to make it more difficult for yourself to succeed?

It's important you do your best, give it your all and put into practice everything that I have said.

Your success will have a positive impact on you and those around you and this is something worth putting effort in for.

This is a long term plan, you can't lose 5 stone without first losing 1 stone and you can't lose 1 stone without losing the very first pound.

Patience and persistence are key to your success. Don't forget, the goal of this is not just to achieve a target weight and then slowly put it all back on again, we are talking long term healthy weight management. No yo-yoing and dieting cycles for you!

Some of the techniques and advice I have given may seem trivial and some may seem like they will have a negligible effect. The true power of this approach is that it encompasses all aspects of your interactions with food, you are making a multi pronged attack on your weight. The combination of techniques and change for you is going to result in big change and big rewards and is far more effective than just making one single change.

Just because something seems like it won't have much impact, does not mean it is not worth doing as it can still be an important part of the process. Even a multi million pound Formula 1 car can be halted by the failure of a 5 pence nut located deep in the engine.

Results will take time, nothing happens overnight and just as your weight gain took months and years, the loss of weight will take time as well. It's really easy to eat 5000 calories in a day, but it will take much longer to lose that amount!

That is why patience is important. If you are doing the right things, the success will come. I've not mentioned anything in this book that is not worth doing, if it wasn't worth doing and did not result in positive outcomes, I would not have included it.

Even if you make all the changes I've talked about, you may not see any results in the first week. Results in the first month could also be not as you expect.

Do you think anyone got anywhere with a million percent effort in the first week and then none after that? You need to put in a good amount of effort on a consistent basis to get those results. It's easy to get demoralised after a week and think that it's not working.

If you make the same changes day after day, week after week, month after month then the results will be incredible. You don't go to work and put in a really good effort for one day and expect promotion or a pay rise. You put in that effort over months and maybe even years to get your reward. Of course, there are setbacks and off days but on average, you've put in enough effort to warrant a reward.

Consistency and perseverance will reward you. It's important that you do persevere, though, because I didn't write this book so someone could lose masses of weight quickly and then slowly put it back on again.

You read this book because you want to be a healthy weight in the long term and because you wanted permanent change. Change doesn't always come easy but if you don't give up and have the right mindset, you will achieve your goals.

You now have the information and the desire to go and

implement changes into your life with the goal of achieving your healthy weight. I know you will succeed because you are prepared to make those changes.

There's a saying in martial arts that a black belt is simply a white belt who did not quit.

If you keep up what you started, your goals will be reached.

I'd love to know how you get on and what your experiences have been on your journey towards your goals. My email address is neil@neilashbyweightloss.co.uk.

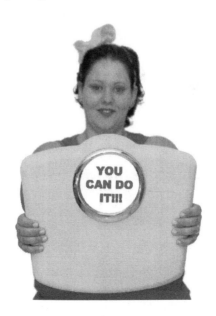

© Depositphotos.com/luislouro

References

Chapter 1 - The Successful Weight Loss Mindset

1.   http://www.patient.co.uk/health/obesity-and-overweight-in-adults

2.http://www.nhs.uk/news/2009/03March/Pages/Obesityincreasesdeathrisk.aspx

3.   http://www.fitnessforweightloss.com/diet-and-weight-loss-statistics/

4.   http://www.femalefirst.co.uk/health/length-of-the-average-diet-279944.html

5.http://www.dailymail.co.uk/femail/article-2204944/Women-spend-staggering-SEVENTEEN-years-lives-trying-lose-weight.html

Chapter 2 - Successful Approaches to Change

1. http://en.wikipedia.org/wiki/Atkins_diet

2.http://www.bda.uk.com/news/121122FadDiets2012.html,
http://www.bda.uk.com/news/111117CelebDiets.html,
http://www.bda.uk.com/news/101213weirddiets.html

3.http://www.dailymail.co.uk/femail/article-2110165/Ketogenic-Enteral-Nutrition-diet-NHS-specialist-recommends-fed-drip-lose-weight.html

Chapter 3 - An Environment for Successful Weight Loss

1. Wansink, "Focus on Nutritional Gatekeepers and the 72% solution", Journal of the America Dietetic Association, September 2006

Chapter 6 - Behaviour for Successful Weight Loss

1. John M. DeCastrp "Eating Behaviour: Lessons from the Real World of Humans", 1994

2.http://www.72point.com/coverage/tv-dinners-60-meals-eaten-front-television/

3. http://www.ncl.ac.uk/press.office/press.release/item/new-regulations-fail-to-make-tv-food-adverts-healthier-for-children

4. http://www.ncbi.nlm.nih.gov/pmc/articles/PMC2743554

/

5.http://stakeholders.ofcom.org.uk/market-data-research/market-data/communications-market-reports/cmr12/tv-audio-visual/uk-2.42/

6.http://www.nationalgrid.com/NR/rdonlyres/1C4B1304-ED58-4631-8A84-3859FB8B4B38/17136/demand.pdf

Chapter 7 - Thursday Big Shop

1.http://www.telegraph.co.uk/finance/newsbysector/retailandconsumer/9907620/Supermarkets-British-shoppers-fatal-attraction.html

http://www.uea.ac.uk/mac/comm/media/press/2012/November/supermarkets-offers-paul-dobson

2.   http://lifehacker.com/5061720/impulse-buys-most-common-at-the-grocery-store

http://www.thesun.co.uk/sol/homepage/news/4638004/Bargain-offers-in-our-main-supermarkets-are-often-fabricated.html

3.
http://foodpsychology.cornell.edu/pdf/permission/1990-2000/Anchoring-JMR-1998.pdf

http://abcnews.go.com/Health/checkout-line-impulse-buys-contribute-obesity/story?id=17446327#.UdwBlU1wZdI

Chapter 8 - Reading Between the Labels

1.http://www.npr.org/blogs/thesalt/2011/12/31/14447
8009/the-average-american-ate-literally-a-ton-this-year

2.
http://facts.randomhistory.com/2008/12/02_nutrition.h
tml

Chapter 9 - Successful Portion Control

1.
http://www.telegraph.co.uk/health/dietandfitness/9335
820/Lose-weight-by-changing-the-colour-of-your-
plate.html

2. http://www.subwaydeliver.co.uk/buildsub.php?id=36

3. Wansink, B. & Payne, C.R. (2007). Counting bones:
Environmental cues that decrease food intake.
Perceptual and Motor Skills - See more at:
http://blog.nasm.org/fitness/mindless-to-mindful-
eating-for-weight-loss/#sthash.Oj7Y8w6E.dpuf

Printed in Great Britain
by Amazon.co.uk, Ltd.,
Marston Gate.